STARK LIBRARY JUN - - 2022

DISCARD

GETTING REAL STRATEGIES FOR TEENS IN NEED

I GET PANIC ATTACKS... WHAT'S NEXT?

VERITY MILLER

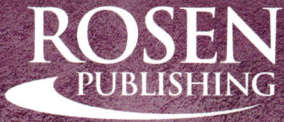
NEW YORK

Published in 2022 by The Rosen Publishing Group, Inc.
29 East 21st Street, New York, NY 10010

Copyright © 2022 by The Rosen Publishing Group, Inc.

First Edition

Designer: Rachel Rising
Editor: Greg Roza

Portions of this work were originally authored by Anne Spencer and published as *I Get Panic Attacks. Now What?* All new material in this edition was authored by Verity Miller.

All rights reserved. No part of this book may be reproduced in any form without permission in writing from the publisher, except by a reviewer.

Library of Congress Cataloging-in-Publication Data
Names: Miller, Verity, author.
Title: I get panic attacks...what's next? / Verity Miller.
Description: New York : Rosen Publishing, 2022. | Series: Getting real: strategies for teens in need | Includes index.
Identifiers: LCCN 2021006999 | ISBN 9781499470604 (library binding) | ISBN 9781499470598 (paperback) | ISBN 9781499470611 (ebook)
Subjects: LCSH: Anxiety in adolescence. | Panic attacks.
Classification: LCC RJ506.A58 M57 2022 | DDC 618.92/8522--dc23
LC record available at https://lccn.loc.gov/2021006999

Some of the images in this book illustrate individuals who are models. The depictions do not imply actual situations or events.

Manufactured in the United States of America

CPSIA Compliance Information: Batch #CSRYA22. For further information contact Rosen Publishing, New York, New York at 1-800-237-9932.

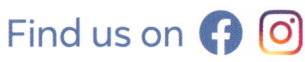

CONTENTS

INTRODUCTION 4

CHAPTER 1
LEARNING ABOUT ANXIETY AND PANIC ATTACKS 8

CHAPTER 2
WHY IS THIS HAPPENING? 18

CHAPTER 3
AN ARRAY OF ANXIETY AND PANIC DISORDERS 34

CHAPTER 4
WHAT CAN YOU DO? 50

CHAPTER 5
MEDICATION MIGHT HELP 70

CHAPTER 6
HOW TO FIND HELP 78

CHAPTER 7
LIVING WITH ANXIETY AND STRESS 86

GLOSSARY 96

FOR MORE INFORMATION 98

FOR FURTHER READING 100

INDEX 102

ABOUT THE AUTHOR 104

INTRODUCTION

Your heart is racing. You're breathing more quickly than usual. Perhaps you can't concentrate, and your muscles are tense. Your stomach hurts. Maybe your hands or legs are shaking.

Could you be having a panic attack?

Everyone panics or feels anxiety sometimes. That's not unusual. Panic and fear can even be good things, because they prepare you to get out of danger or deal with situations that could hurt you. But when you're anxious most of the time for no real reason or often get feelings of panic you can't control or don't understand, it's time to consider talking to someone else and investigating if you might be having panic attacks.

Panic attacks are a type of anxiety disorder, a mental health condition that involves more anxiety, fear, or worry than is usual. Many people have anxiety disorders, and they're nothing to be ashamed of. They can affect people of all ages, and they can start at any age. Sometimes they start slowly and gradually, and sometimes they start all at once. Someone who has repeated panic attacks without a specific trigger may have an anxiety disorder called panic disorder.

While panic disorder and other anxiety disorders are mental health conditions, they can have physical signs and symptoms. If your brain is tell-

INTRODUCTION | 5

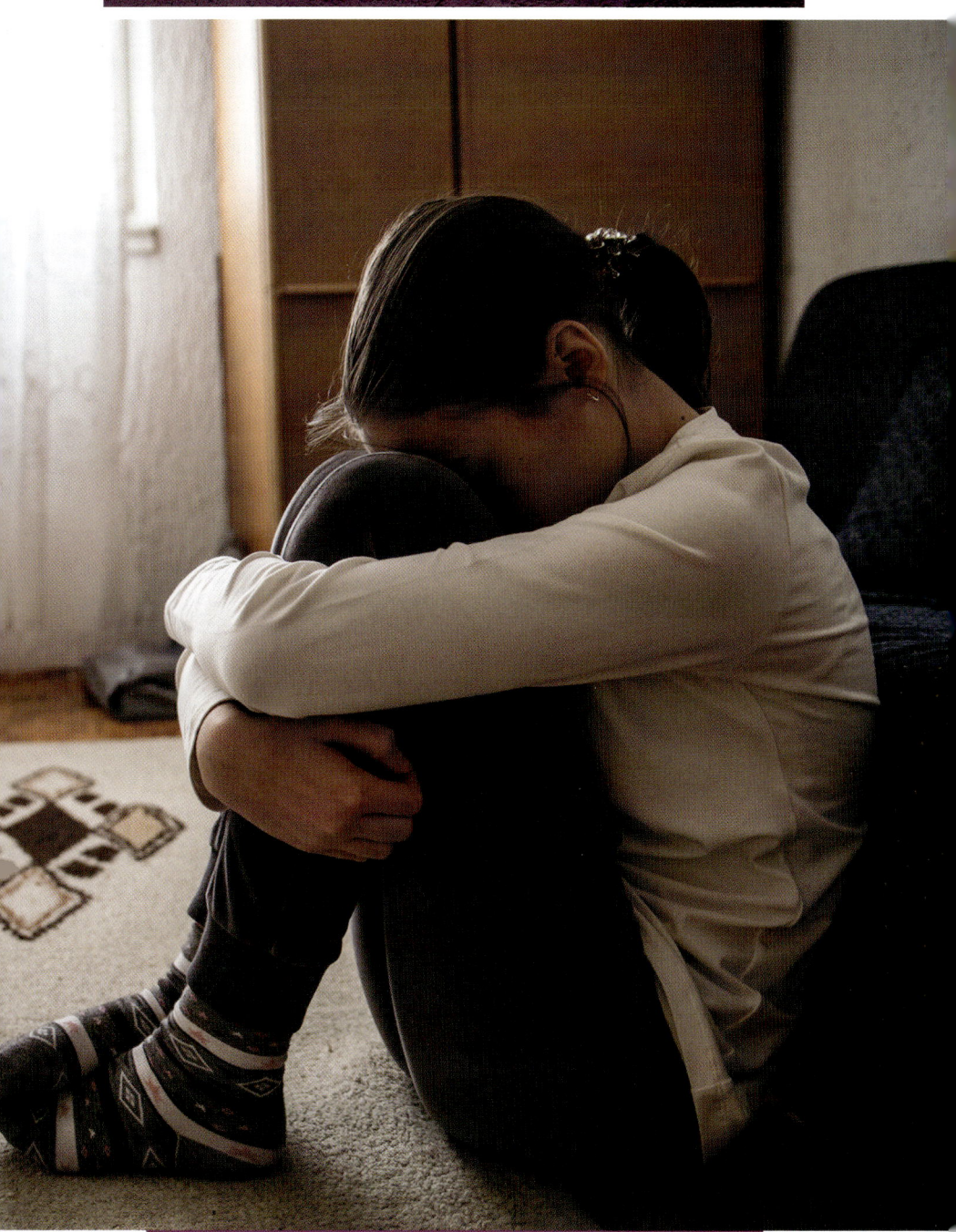

Panic attacks can be scary. You may think something is seriously wrong and there's nothing that can help. However, there are ways you can manage anxiety and panic and make things better.

ing your body there's reason to panic, your body will be on high alert even when there's no actual reason. You might be tense a lot, which can cause injury and pain. This constant state of alert can weaken your immune system and make you more likely to get sick. You may also have more stomach issues, including ulcers and irritable bowel syndrome.

More than 40 million adults in the United States have some sort of anxiety disorder, and about 2.4 million of them have panic disorder. About half of them developed these anxiety disorders before they were 21 years old. In addition, about 7 percent of young people ages 3 to 17 have issues with anxiety each year.

You're not alone. And you can fight back against panic attacks and anxiety disorders in many ways. Keep reading to learn more.

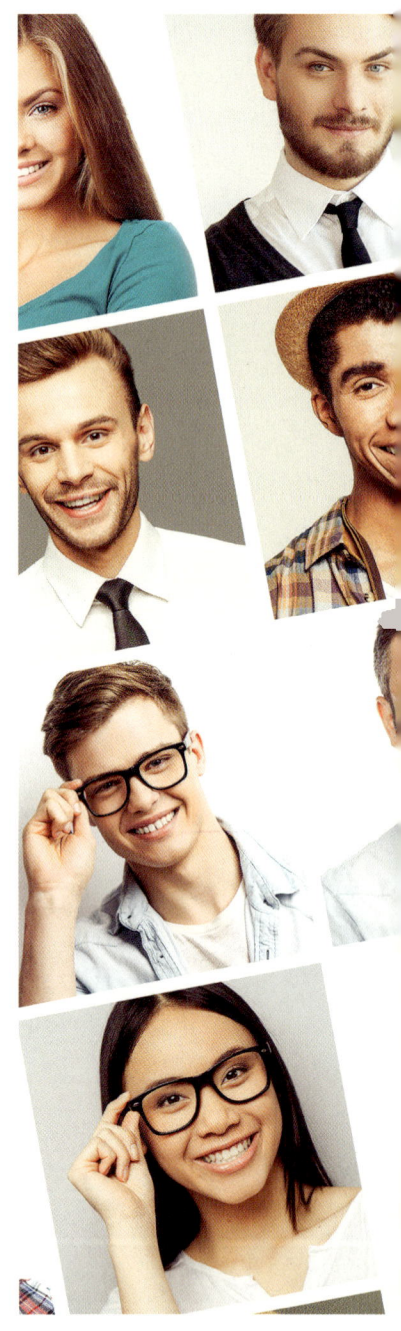

INTRODUCTION 7

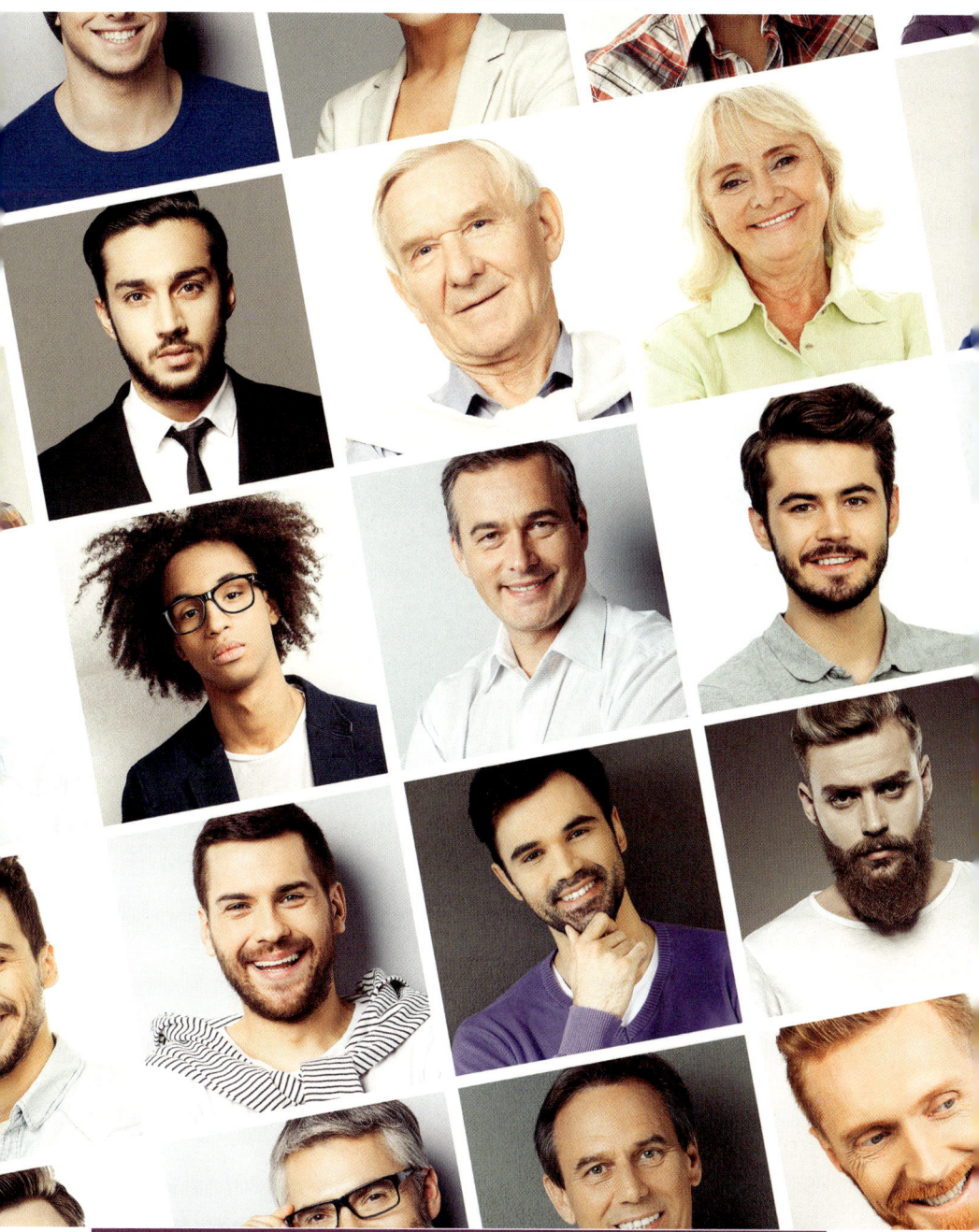

Any one of these people could have a panic disorder. In fact, some of them almost certainly do! It's nothing to be embarrassed of, and there's help out there.

CHAPTER 1

LEARNING ABOUT ANXIETY AND PANIC ATTACKS

So what, precisely, does a panic attack feel like?

A panic attack is an episode of intense fear with no immediate apparent cause. It includes related physical symptoms such as feeling like your heart is pounding or like you can't breathe. It can make you feel like you're dying even when you're in no danger at all. It can happen in the middle of the night or when you're in school, out of nowhere. It can be terrifying!

A panic attack usually has at least four of these symptoms: chest pain or discomfort, fast heart rate or a feeling of pounding, shaking, sweating, shortness of breath, feeling like you're choking, chills or hot flashes, nausea or stomach pain, feeling dizzy or faint, numbness, a feeling of distance from reality, fear of dying, or fear of losing control. They usually come on quickly and peak in 10 minutes or so.

LEARNING ABOUT ANXIETY AND PANIC ATTACKS

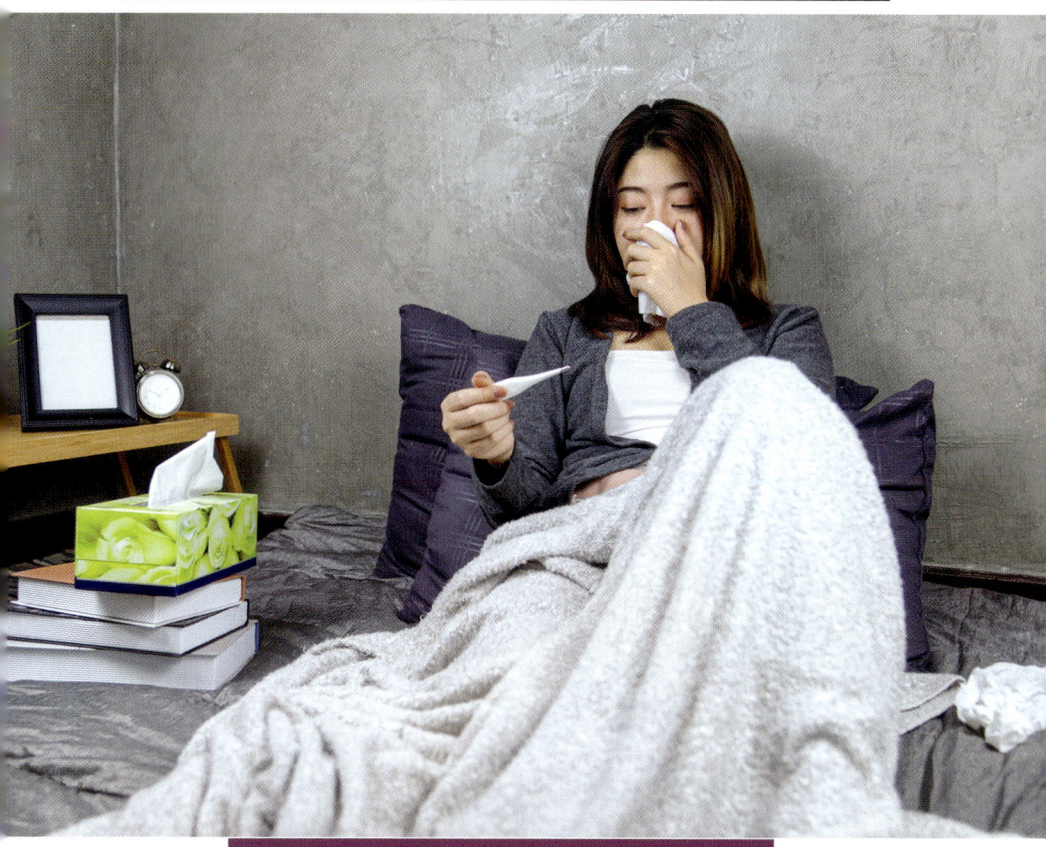

Panic attacks can make you believe that you're sick—or that you're dying. But they can't really hurt you.

Many people have one or two panic attacks in their lifetime. This doesn't mean they have panic disorder. Other people have panic attacks caused by other anxiety disorders. These are usually caused by specific triggers. Those with panic disorder will spend a lot of time worrying about another attack, maybe even changing their behavior to try to avoid one.

It's important to know that anxiety and panic attacks aren't just all in your head. They can be caused by very real physical phenomena. Scientists don't understand all the physical causes for anxiety disorders yet, but there are a few that are widely accepted.

Sometimes brain biochemistry can be at fault. People may have an imbalance in a neurotransmitter—a chemical messenger in the brain. Neurotransmitters include serotonin, dopamine, norepinephrine, and gamma-aminobutyric acid (GABA). Low levels of serotonin may cause depression or anxiety, while dopamine can have an effect on a person's energy levels and more. Norepinephrine is released during the body's reaction to stress and can cause a "flight or fight" reaction. Gamma-aminobutyric acid

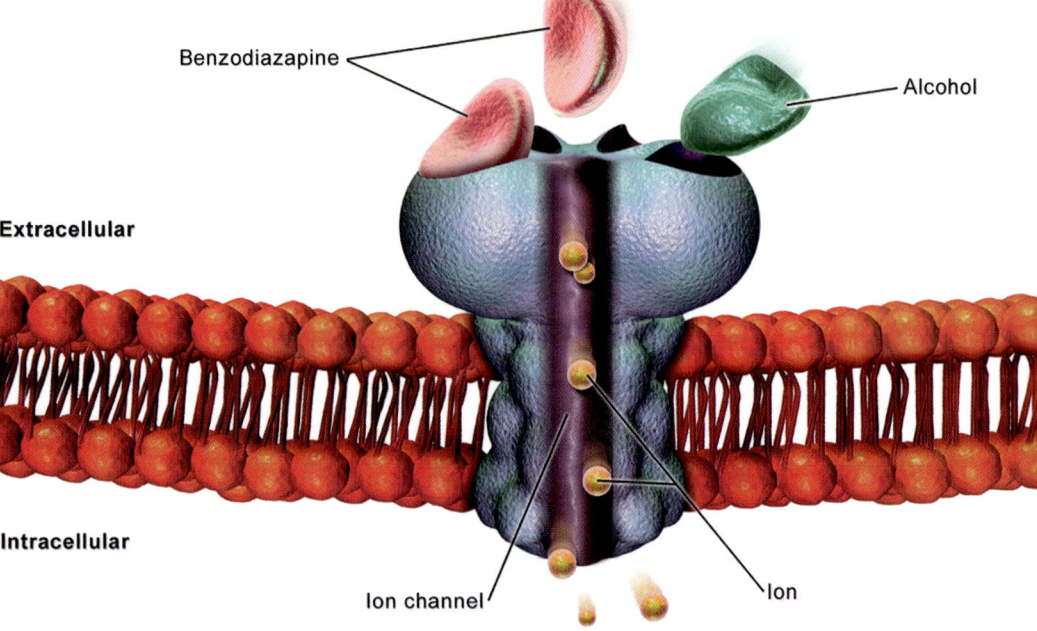

This diagram shows that a GABA's effect can be heightened by alcohol and some drugs. Benzodiazepines are drugs that calm the nerves, sometimes called tranquilizers. Never take a drug unless it's been prescribed for you.

AGORAPHOBIA

People who have panic attacks often begin to worry a great deal about whether (or when) they'll have another one. This is a hallmark of panic disorder. This worry may cause them to avoid places where they think a panic attack might take place or avoid situations or circumstances they associate with a panic attack. Often, they avoid places that would be particularly embarrassing or difficult to get out of if a panic attack happens.

Sometimes, this fear and worry become so strong that the person avoids going anywhere they think a panic attack might happen. This is called agoraphobia. In some cases, a person with agoraphobia avoids places such as a mall or normal activities such as driving. They may need someone else to be with them before they do certain things. Sometimes, the condition becomes so strong that they avoid leaving their home altogether.

About one-third of people with a panic disorder will develop agoraphobia. However, early treatment of panic disorder can help prevent this. Children and teens can develop agoraphobia too. This can lead to avoiding places such as school or situations such as social activities or being in a school bus. More girls than boys tend to develop agoraphobia, just like more girls than boys tend to develop panic attacks.

calms the brain, so low levels of this neurotransmitter may cause high anxiety.

Genetics may also have a lot to do with panic disorders. If someone in your family has such a disorder, you're at higher risk for developing one too.

This might have to do with neurotransmitters such as those discussed above. Panic disorders do tend to run in families. Some medical conditions, including endocrine disorders such as hypoglycemia and some thyroid disorders, also cause heightened anxiety.

However, outside forces can also affect anxiety. Some drugs, including caffeine, nicotine, and illegal drugs such as amphetamines and cocaine, can all cause anxiety. Some medications can also cause or heighten anxiety.

SLEEP ISSUES

Panic attacks can affect many parts of your life, including your sleep. It may not be uncommon for an attack to wake you up at night—and then the lingering symptoms may keep you awake for even longer, even if the attack itself was only minutes long. That can wreak havoc with your sleep schedule.

People with anxiety disorders, such as panic attacks, often have sleep issues such as insomnia. Worries, especially obsessive ones, can make it tough to shut off your brain and settle down. And once you've had a nighttime panic attack, the worry about having another one can keep you up.

Unfortunately, a lack of sleep can cause anxiety to get worse—so it's even more important to find ways to cope with symptoms that can keep you up at night before the situation turns into a vicious cycle. Other conditions, such as sleep apnea, can also cause nighttime panic attacks. And nightmares, though

LEARNING ABOUT ANXIETY AND PANIC ATTACKS   13

not panic attacks, can cause issues. So can night terrors. (Some sources consider night terrors to be

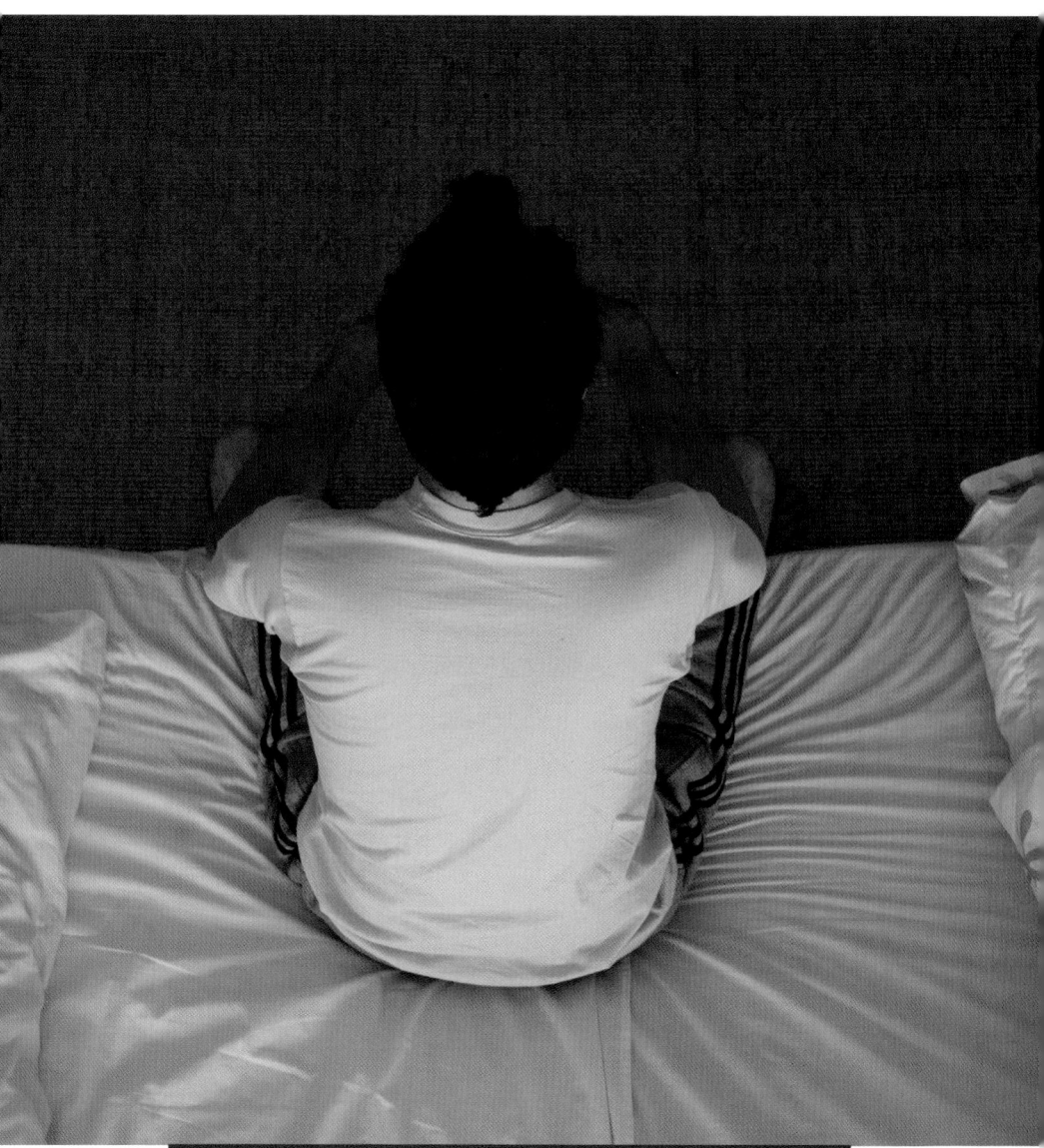

The more tired you get, the more difficult it is to keep anxiety under control. Anxiety then keeps you from falling asleep. It's an awful cycle.

nocturnal panic attacks, while others consider them to be a separate thing.

Nightmares and night terrors are both linked to anxiety, but they occur during different levels of sleep. When you fall asleep, your body goes through four levels of sleep. Stage I is the lightest level of sleep; stage IV is the deepest and most restorative to the body. After you have been in stage IV sleep for about 30 minutes, you start to rouse from this deep state and slip back into a lighter sleep. You go up through stage III to stage II sleep.

This cycle happens throughout the night. These four stages of sleep make up NREM (non-rapid eye movement) sleep, during which people don't usually dream. You pass through each night drifting in and out of stages II and III, spending less and less time in stage IV.

Between the stages is another kind of sleep: REM (rapid eye movement) sleep. This is when you dream. REM sleep is believed to be mentally restorative; without it, you would be edgy and irritable all the time. The REM periods get longer throughout the night. By morning, you're spending much more time in REM.

Nightmares occur during REM sleep, so they frequently occur later in the sleep cycle. Nightmares happen more often to people who are under a lot of stress or have suffered trauma, because they're using all their energy during the day to keep thoughts of the trauma at bay. When they fall asleep, their guard is down. Memories come back in the form of bad dreams.

Night terrors, which affect about 40 percent of children and fewer adults, happen during NREM sleep. They're not dreams—at least not the type of dream with a storyline. When someone is in stage IV sleep, they're very relaxed. If someone tried to wake the person, it would be difficult. As they return to the lighter stage III sleep, they sometimes have difficulty

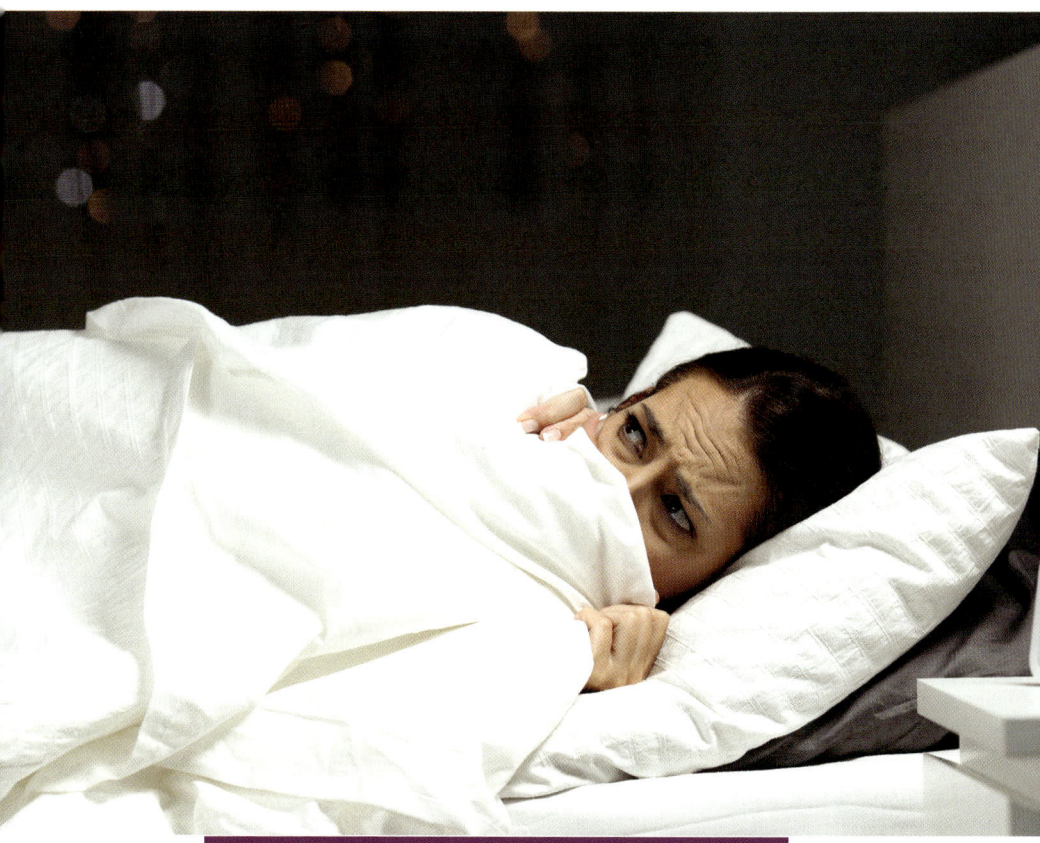

A lack of sleep can make anxiety worse. But what do you do when it's anxiety that makes you unable to fall asleep?

making the transition. If the person is overtired or under a lot of stress, their body may resist coming out of stage IV, and they wake up—but they just appear to be awake. They remember any scary image or thought that preceded this waking up, and they may scream in terror. They may thrash around or fall off the bed. If you try to calm a person who has had a night terror, you may only succeed in scaring them more because they don't know where they are or who you are. In the morning, they likely won't remember the event at all.

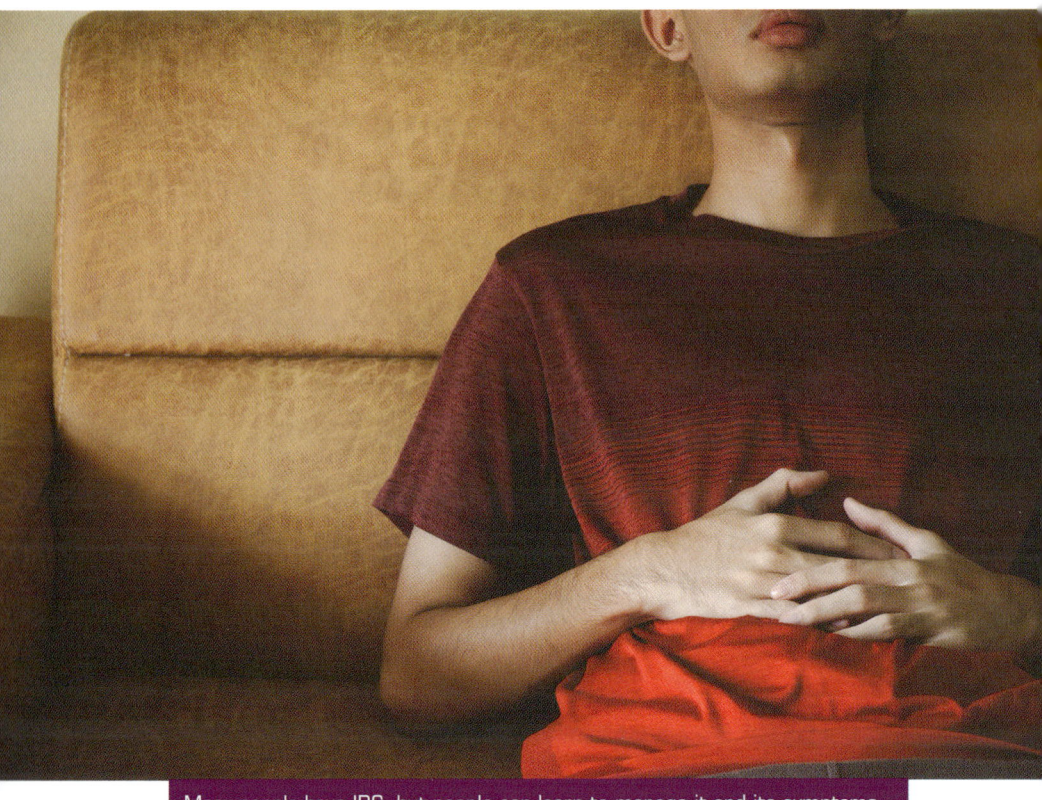

Many people have IBS, but people can learn to manage it and its symptoms.

STOMACH ISSUES AND IBS

Irritable bowel syndrome is a gastrointestinal disorder that affects the colon and the digestive system. Many people who have IBS also deal with panic attacks or other anxiety disorders, and vice versa, although no one's quite sure why the connection exists. It might have something to do with an overactive flight-or-fight response. If you have panic attacks, you might want to watch for signs of IBS as well.

Symptoms of IBS include abdominal pain, stomachaches, cramps, changes in bowel movements from diarrhea to constipation, and bloating and extra gas. Sometimes the two disorders also go hand in hand because both can cause people to avoid certain situations and places due to worry about an attack.

LEARNING TO COPE

Panic attacks can be a horrible experience. They can lead people to believe that they're dying or that something is very wrong with them. However, panic attacks can't actually hurt you. They're not a heart attack, and they're not a stroke. You can learn to deal with them and to live with them.

However, the worry and anxiety that come with panic attacks can wear you down and damage your immune system. They can be damaging to your mental health and overall well-being. They can hurt relationships with friends and family and keep you from doing things you used to love. That's why it's so important to take steps to treat panic disorder and anxiety.

CHAPTER 2

WHY IS THIS HAPPENING?

Often, panic attacks result from a combination of emotional and physical factors, with one setting off the other. Danger activates the fight-or-flight response in the human brain. Things can go wrong, however. Any malfunction in the brain, especially in the region of the lower brain called the locus coeruleus (which controls emotional responses), can cause panic symptoms. Scientists have discovered that they can induce panic symptoms by stimulating this region electrically.

Several different situations can set off panic symptoms in the locus coeruleus. If you're extremely sensitive to carbon dioxide, you may react with panic symptoms when too much carbon dioxide is in your body. This may happen because of hyperventilation—breathing too fast and too shallowly. People who are anxious tend to hyperventilate, and hyperventilating leads to a buildup of carbon dioxide circulating in the system. Carbon dioxide buildup also may happen after exercise.

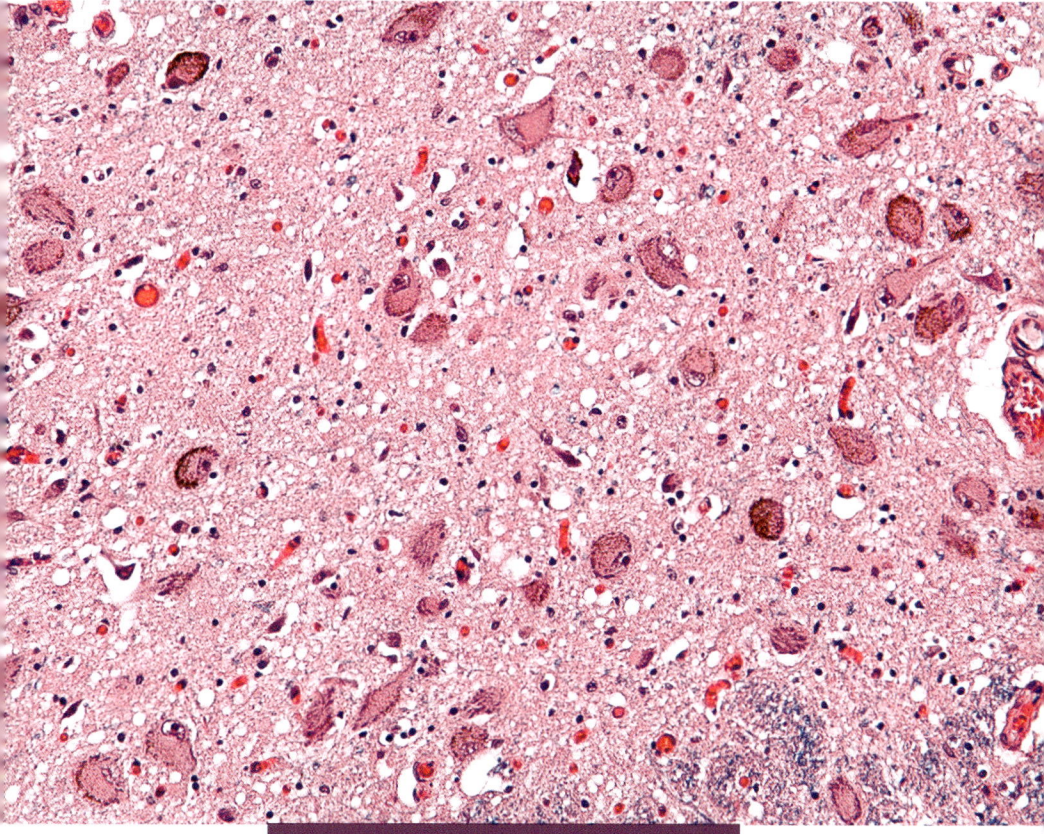

The locus coeruleus is located in the brainstem. This photo shows a highly magnified view of it.

There is a connection between the locus coeruleus and the quantity of neurotransmitters in that region as well. Sometimes too few or too many neurotransmitters (in this case, norepinephrine and serotonin) cause the locus coeruleus to go haywire. This sets off a panic attack. That is why certain antidepressant medications that directly affect the quantity of norepinephrine and serotonin help to prevent panic attacks.

PANIC ATTACKS AND OCD
Obsessive-compulsive disorder (OCD) is a mental health condition that causes repeated unwanted thoughts or feelings or the urge to do something over and over again. While everyone has thoughts that repeat sometimes or particular ways of doing things, people with OCD have obsessions or compulsions that take hours a day, are out of their control, aren't enjoyable, or interfere with their lives.

Doctors have recognized that people with obsessive-compulsive disorder may have a chemical imbalance. They may suffer from unusually low levels of the neurotransmitter serotonin. Serotonin affects memory, sleep, appetite, mood, and the ability to keep from doing repetitive actions. Medications known to increase levels of serotonin may allow someone dealing with obsessive-compulsive disorder to manage it in better ways.

ANXIETY AS A RESULT OF STRESS
Although there's a physiological basis for many panic attacks, as well as a possible genetic component (because anxiety disorders tend to run in families), other factors, such as stress and how a person reacts to stress, play a role.

Sometimes the way people react to stressful situations causes them to develop symptoms of anxiety. If, say, you work at a job that gives you more than one person can reasonably do, you may feel stress as you try to keep up, especially if you're concerned your

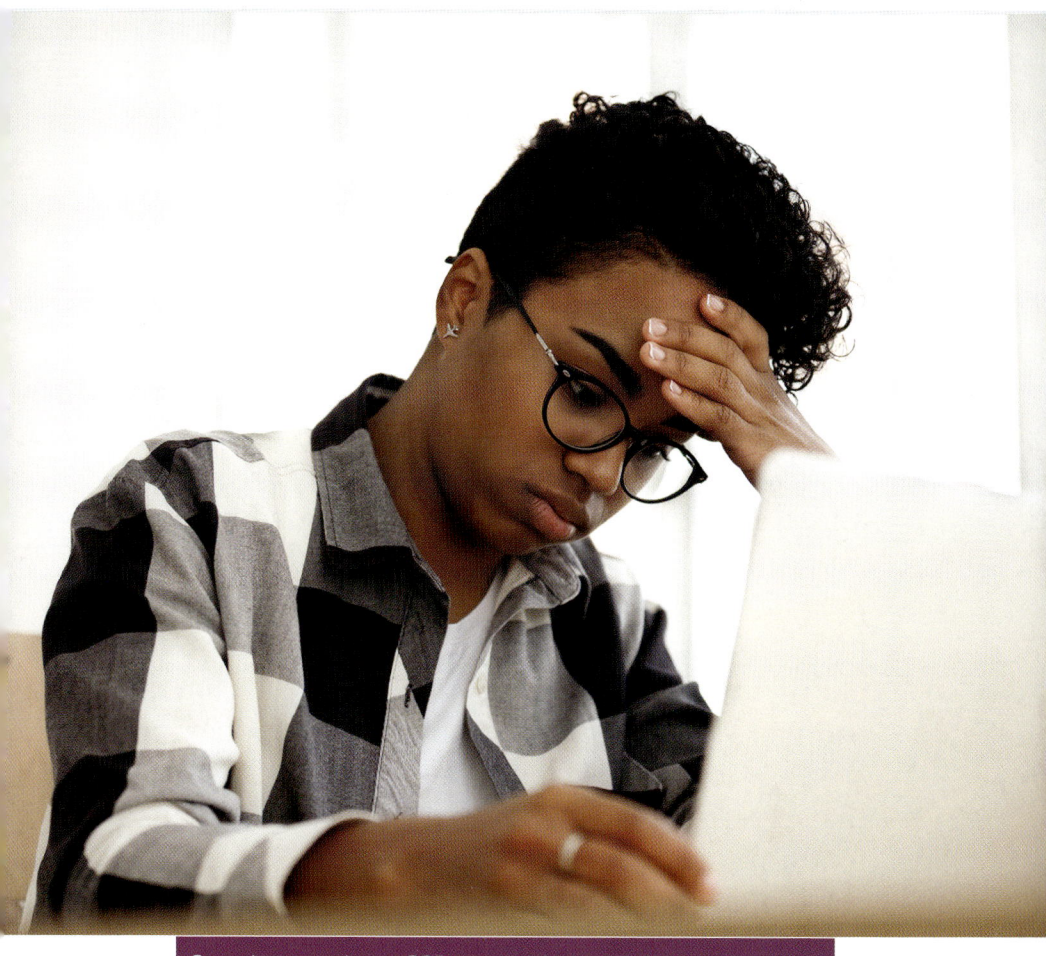

Sometimes people use OCD as a bit of a joke. They'll say things like "Oh, I like things just so! I'm so OCD!" This isn't really funny. OCD is no joke to those who have to cope with it.

boss will get rid of you if you protest or complain and if you really need the job. You'd probably feel pretty anxious at the idea of going back to that job day after day!

However, while stressful situations contribute to anxiety, if people learn to deal effectively with them, they don't have to let their symptoms of anxiety turn into full-fledged anxiety disorders. People can learn ways to stand up for themselves, set boundaries, and manage their feelings.

ANXIETY AS A RESULT OF TRAUMA

Some doctors believe that trauma causes biological changes within the brain, and there's some evidence for this. Trauma can also work on an emotional level to cause anxiety and panic.

Think of someone whose home was wiped out by a tornado while they hid in their basement. Now, every time there's a storm, and the sky gets dark, they have a panic attack. Their original panic, the night the disaster happened, was based on reality, but their continuing panic attacks are based on the trauma. Most storms don't turn into tornadoes, but it's easy to see how someone who's been through that experience might have a strong panic response to a storm.

Another example could be someone who was bitten by a dog as a child and is terrified by all dogs even as an adult. They could still have this response around friendly dogs that wouldn't harm them. Their panic is rooted in the trauma of the original experience.

About 20 percent of people who go through serious trauma develop post-traumatic stress disorder (PTSD). Like panic disorder and other mental health conditions, there are treatments for PTSD.

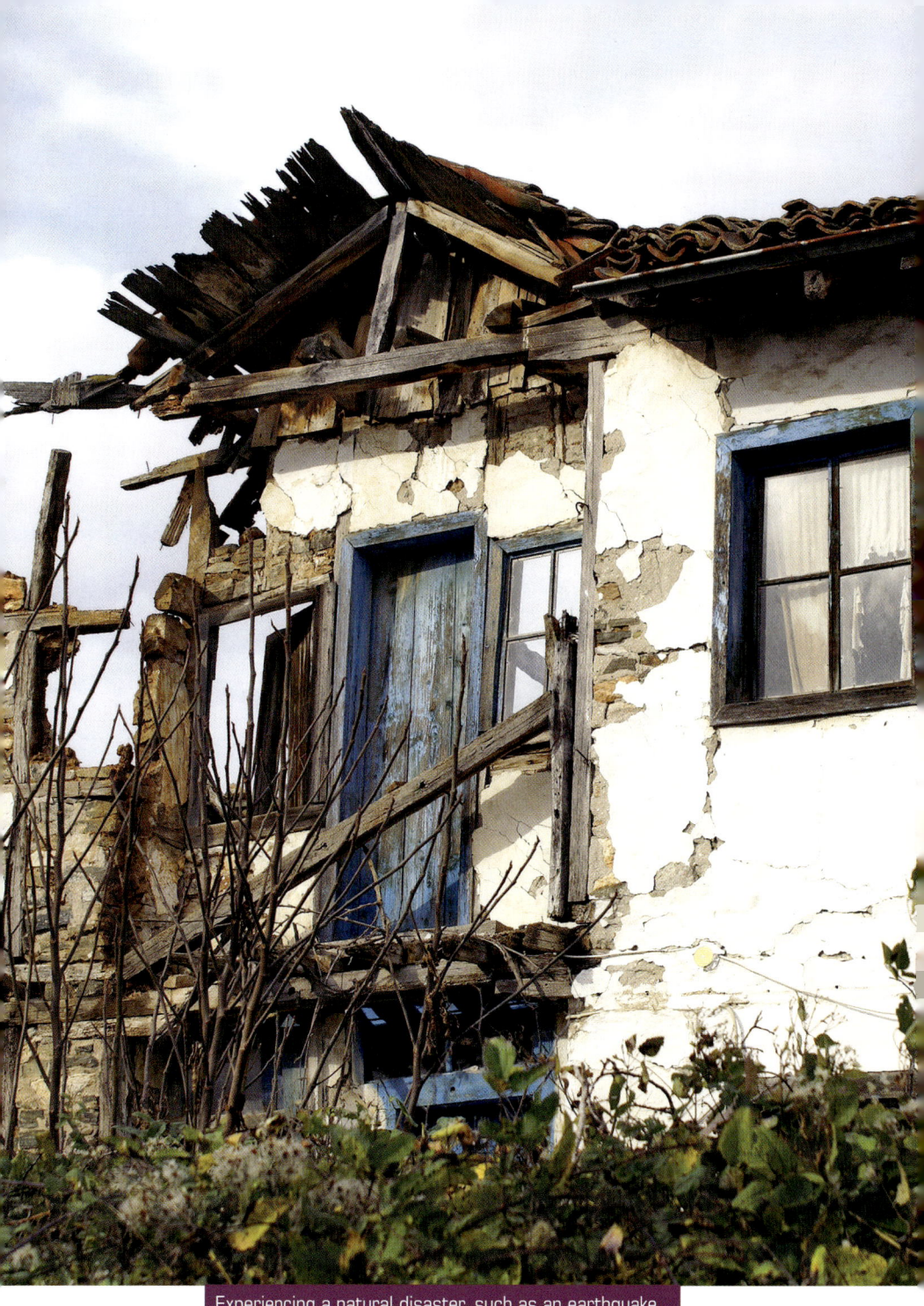

Experiencing a natural disaster, such as an earthquake, can lead to trauma and panic attacks.

MORE ABOUT PTSD

When many people think about post-traumatic stress disorder, they think of military veterans. But while many combat veterans do deal with PTSD, the disorder can affect many different people for many different reasons. Going through or witnessing a traumatic event such as a natural disaster, a serious accident, a terrorist act, or a sexual attack can cause PTSD, as can being a victim of serious threats.

Those who deal with PTSD may have flashbacks, nightmares, and uncontrollable thoughts. Similar to those with other anxiety disorders, they may avoid things, people, and places that they associate with the traumatic event.

People from some ethnic groups, including American Indians, U.S. Latinos, and African Americans, deal with PTSD at a greater rate than others. More women than men are diagnosed with it.

ANXIETY AS A RESULT OF PHOBIAS

A phobia can also cause panic attacks, though the two are ultimately separate anxiety disorders. These strong, uncontrollable fears can lead people to stay away from any situation where they could encounter the thing they fear, whether it's spiders, snakes, close spaces, heights, or needles. A person can also have a social phobia, in which they have an overwhelming fear of being embarrassed or judged badly in a social situation. Agoraphobia is also a phobia, as the name suggests. As with other anxiety disorders, phobias can be managed and treated.

Some scientists think there may be a scientific reason why many people have phobias about snakes and spiders. Since some snakes and spiders are poisonous, they believe that we may be "programmed" to fear them. In earlier times, panicking and running away from snakes may have saved many lives. Unfortunately, even today some people still deal with strong fear even when faced with a harmless garter snake or spider. They react with panic without first assessing the danger.

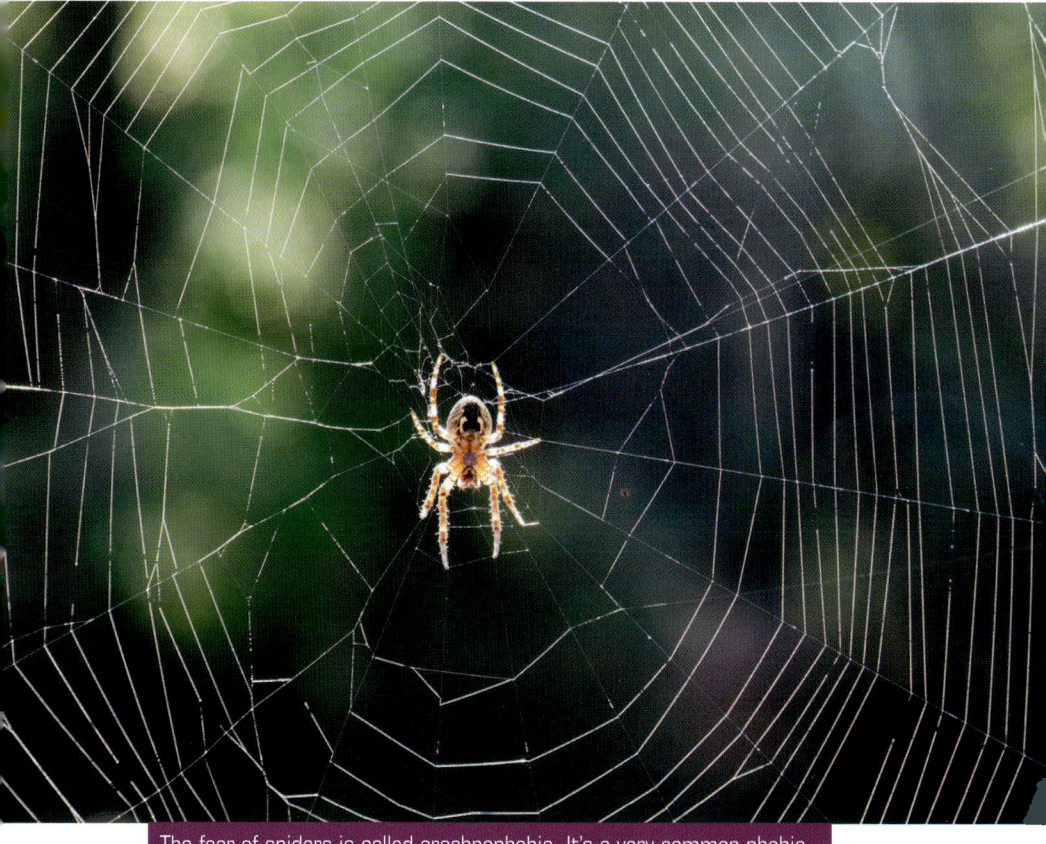

The fear of spiders is called arachnophobia. It's a very common phobia.

NO LAUGHING MATTER

It's probably easy to guess what the most common phobia in the United States is. It's arachnophobia, the fear of spiders! About 30.5 percent of the U.S. population has some level of this phobia. It's followed by ophidiophobia (fear of snakes), acrophobia (fear of heights), aerophobia (fear of flying), cynophobia (fear of dogs), astraphobia (fear of thunder and lightning), trypanophobia (fear of injections), social phobia, agoraphobia, and mysophobia (fear of germs). Other common phobias are claustrophobia (fear of small spaces) and glossophobia (fear of public speaking).

Sometimes people make fun of phobias or say that they have one when they really just have a more low-key dislike or fear of something. To be a phobia, a fear must be so intense and strong that it interferes with their everyday life. Phobias may not be based in logic, but they're no joke. Teasing someone about a true phobia can make the anxiety much worse and make it more likely that they won't seek help for their disorder.

Almost anything can become a phobia. Some of the less well-known ones are arithmophobia (fear of numbers), podophobia (fear of feet), selenophobia (fear of the moon), and ephebiphobia (fear of teenagers).

THE ISSUE OF ANTICIPATION

True panic attacks come from out of the blue. There are often biological reasons for them. But because the symptoms are so frightening, and the events are so unpredictable, the person having the attack may begin to fear having another one. The way they feel—nervous, sweaty palms, stomach tied in knots—is called anticipatory anxiety. In other words, they anticipate having another panic attack at any moment and are constantly on guard. Medication may help keep panic attacks from occurring, but it likely does little to stop the buildup of anxiety.

Anticipatory anxiety comes from not knowing how to deal with the panic situation. People may talk themselves into a worse reaction or rely on other people or substances to make them feel safe. Let's look at some of the ways we make small problems bigger.

Avoidance can be one of the quickest ways to convert a fear into a phobia. Whether a person has been traumatized or associates their first panic attack with a specific situation, once they start avoiding those situations, they may make the fear worse because they haven't faced it. If they change their lifestyle to accommodate the fear, they've created a phobia. So, whether or not a phobia has a biological basis, emotional factors (the way a person thinks about the event and the subsequent way they behave) maintain the phobia.

Some people have another method of handling stressful situations, though it's not a healthy one. When they start feeling anxious, they turn to substances such as drugs and alcohol. Some people start drinking alcohol because they're afraid of social encounters. Fearing a situation in which they might have a panic attack, a person may rely on a substance—such as alcohol, tranquilizers, or illegal drugs—or another person to get them through the situation. If they do this often enough, they associate relief from anxiety with taking the drug or having that particular person with them. Soon enough, they become unable to face the situation without the drug or the person to serve as a safety net. Reliance

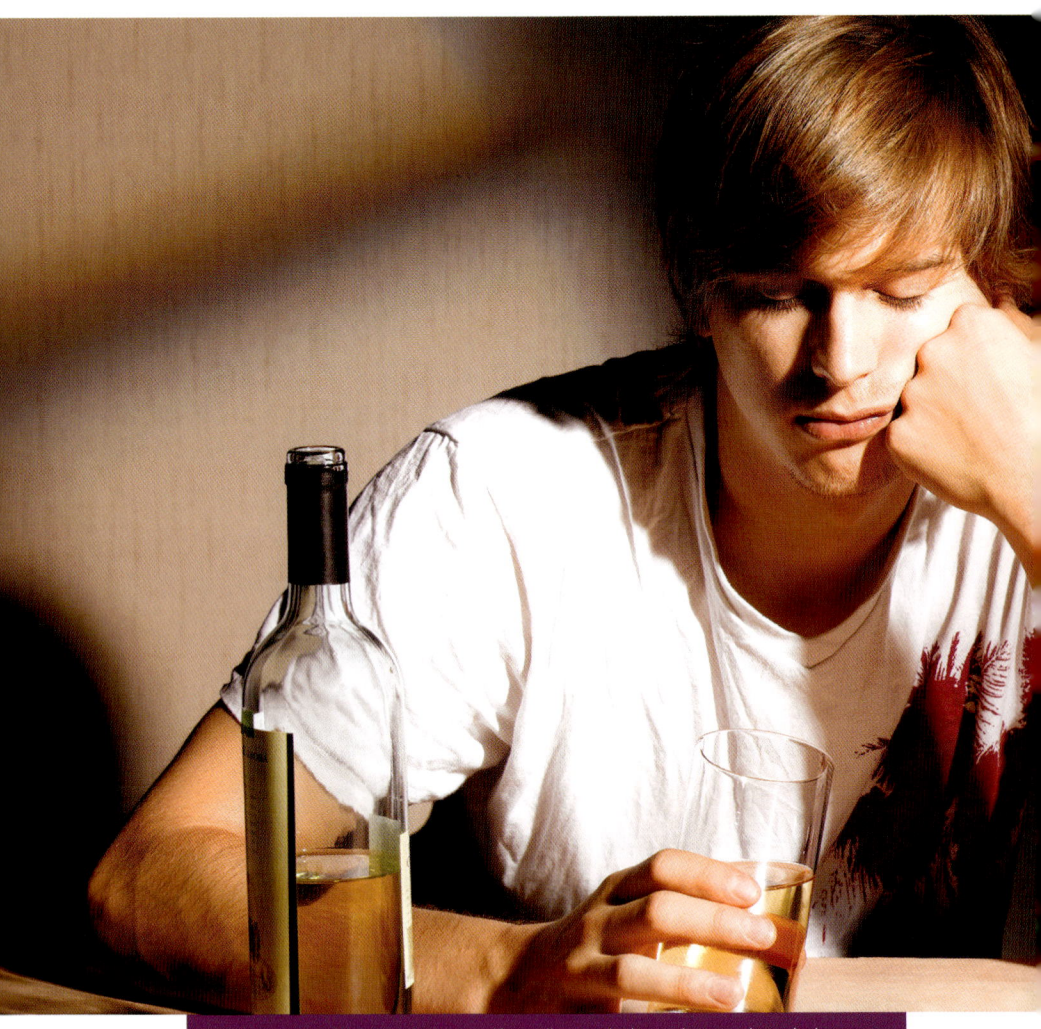

Some people drink alcohol to self-medicate their anxiety and panic issues, but this doesn't work well and is a very unhealthy way of handling it.

on safety nets works the same way as avoidance. Avoiding the source of your fears brings relief, so avoidance becomes a way of life. Likewise, turning to drugs can become a way of life because initially it brings relief from the fear. In addition, having a safety net becomes problematic because you learn you can't handle the situation alone.

This can also lead to drug addiction or alcoholism. Teens can especially get into trouble if they start drinking or using drugs at an early age.

TALKING YOURSELF INTO ANXIETY

Panic attacks are no fun, but sometimes people unintentionally talk themselves into them. This self-talk (what you tell yourself about a situation) can also make a panic attack worse. A person who convinces themselves that they're having a heart attack or a serious medical incident might make the panic attack situation far worse and longer lasting with their own negative thoughts.

30 | I GET PANIC ATTACKS...WHAT'S NEXT?

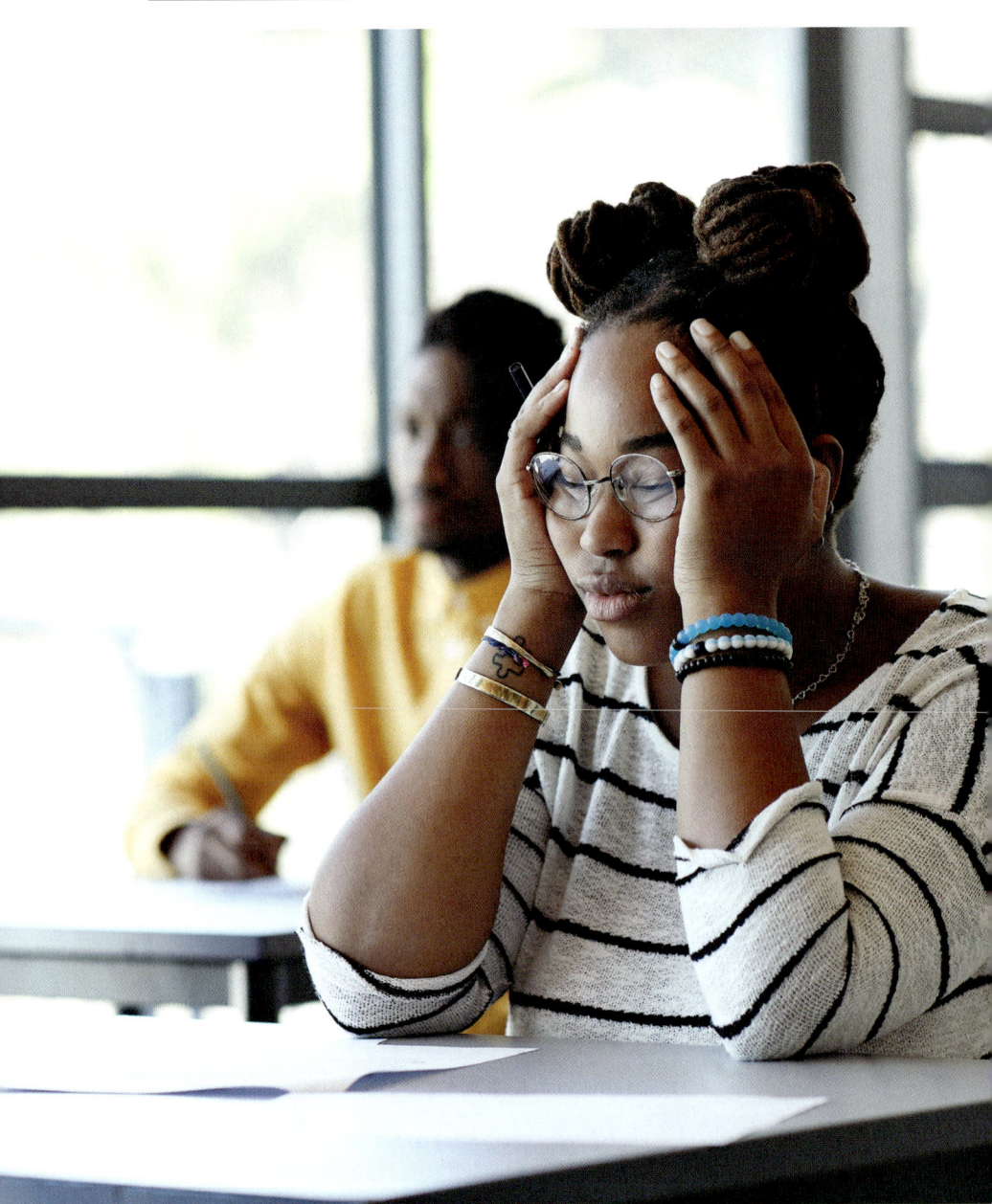

Panic attacks can hit at any time: at home, in school, or in the car. It's important to learn how to deal with them.

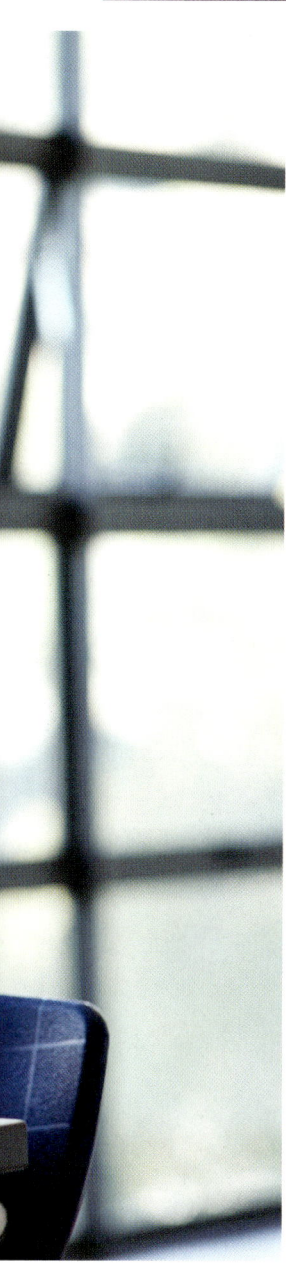

Panic attacks can be scary, but there are ways to talk yourself into riding out the symptoms and getting through them. With negative thoughts—whether those caused by worrying about a serious issue, the reactions of other people, feelings of failure, or other bad things—the panic and anxiety just get worse and last longer. Some kinds of harmful self-talk include focusing on the negative, trying to hold yourself up to an unrealistic ideal, overgeneralizing about negative things ("I'll never figure this out," etc.), all-or-nothing thinking (thinking one negative thing negates all good things), and catastrophic thinking, which is assuming the worst will happen.

There are ways to combat negative thoughts, however. You can learn to recognize them and learn ways to counter them. Positive self-talk, meanwhile, can be a good thing for those with anxiety.

NOT YOUR FAULT

There are many possible underlying cases and reasons for anxiety and panic attacks, and there are many things that can make them worse.

However, there's one very important thing to remember about them: panic attacks are not your fault. You did nothing to deserve them. You don't deserve an anxiety disorder, and you didn't do anything to cause it. It doesn't make you a bad person, and it doesn't make you weak. It doesn't mean there's something wrong with you.

Even if friends and loved ones don't understand what's going on with you, it's key to keep this in mind. Accepting your anxiety disorder may be the first step toward learning how to live with it and work against it. You're not weak for living with a panic disorder—you're very strong!

10 GREAT QUESTIONS TO ASK YOUR DOCTOR

1. What is causing me to have panic attacks and anxiety?
2. How can we treat my panic disorder?
3. Will I have panic attacks my entire life?
4. Do a lot of people deal with panic disorder?
5. Would I be weak if I take medication to help manage my anxiety?
6. Do a lot of people my age have this issue?
7. Are there any day-to-day things about my life that I can change to reduce my panic attacks?
8. Do anxiety medications have many side effects?
9. What should I do in case of an emergency, like an anxiety attack I can't shake?
10. If I talk to you or a therapist about my panic attacks, is what I say confidential?

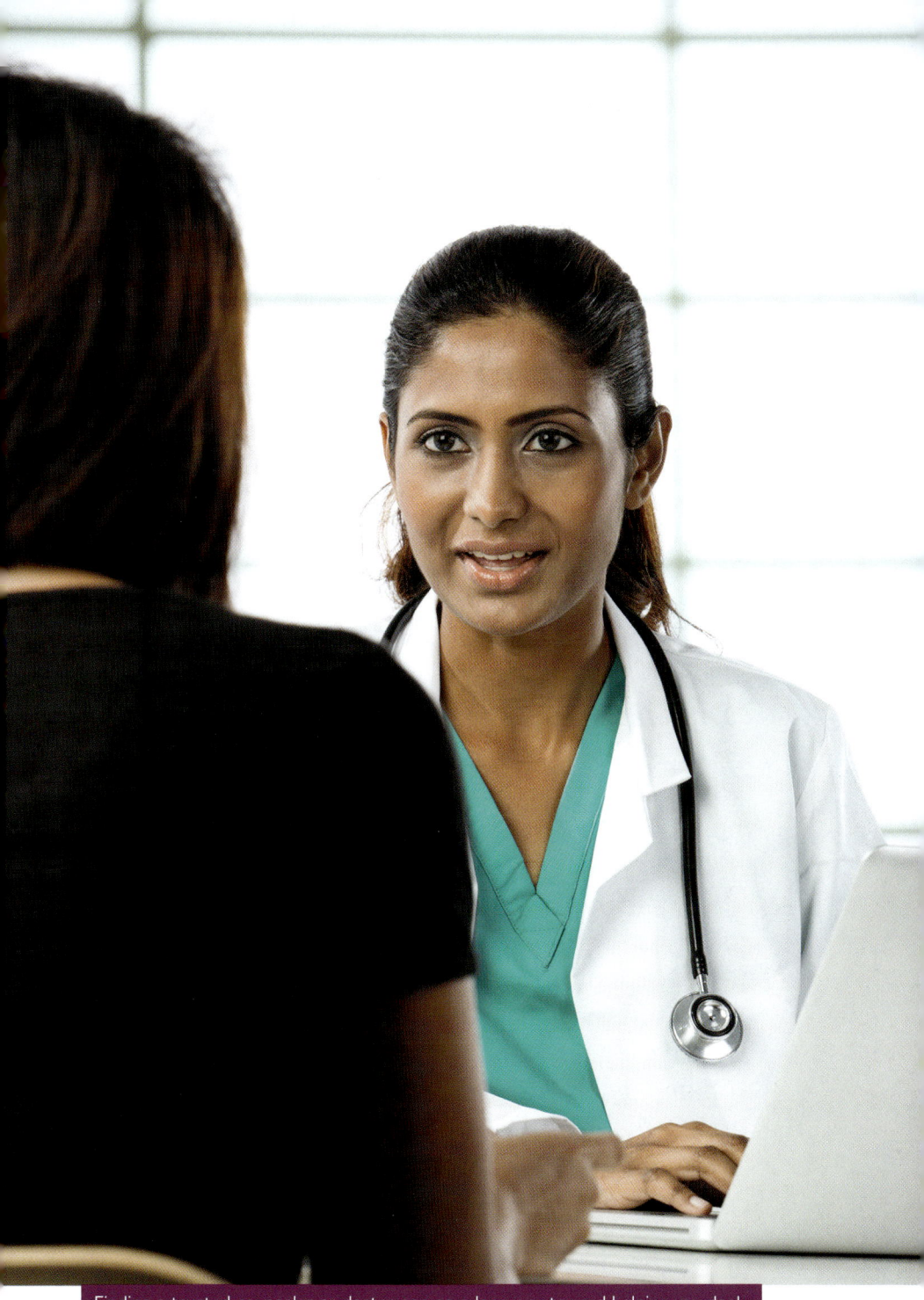

Finding a trusted counselor or doctor can go a long way toward helping you deal with your panic attacks and anxiety. You have to be honest with them, however.

CHAPTER 3

AN ARRAY OF ANXIETY AND PANIC DISORDERS

As of 2021, according to the National Alliance on Mental Illness, more than 40 million Americans suffer from some type of anxiety disorder. These disorders are the most common type of mental health disorder in the United States. While they're quite treatable, however, only about 40 percent of those dealing with these disorders get treatment.

As stated previously, there are many kinds in additional to panic disorder, including generalized anxiety disorder (GAD), in which the person experiences extreme chronic anxiety; social anxiety disorder; phobias; OCD; PTSD; and others. Panic attacks can take place with these disorders in additional to panic disorder, and depression is also linked to anxiety disorders.

THE MOST COMMON ANXIETY DISORDER

Generalized anxiety disorder is the most common sort of anxiety disorder, especially in adults. It often coexists with major depression. GAD signs include persistent, excessive worry about many different things. While some anxiety and worry are a normal part of life, people with this condition often expect disaster and cannot control their worry, even when it's about normal, everyday things such as a job, family, or health.

Doctors usually diagnose it when someone has trouble controlling their worry on more days than not for at least six months. They also would have

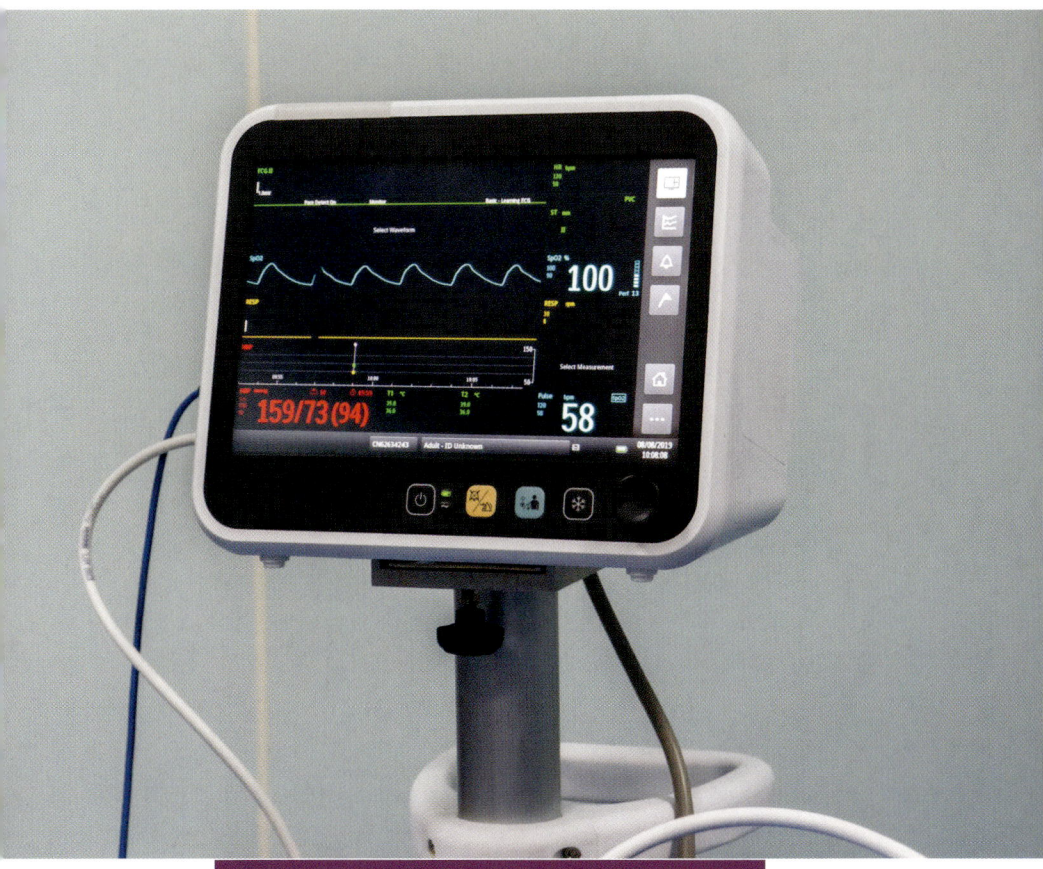

A rapid heartbeat is a sign of a panic attack. Sometimes people mistake this for a heart attack.

three or more symptoms, including an impending sense of doom or danger; feeling nervous or on edge; trouble concentrating; trouble sleeping; increased heart rate; rapid breathing, shaking, or sweating; stomach or gastrointestinal issues; and feelings of weakness or tiredness.

GAD involves three main reactions: physiological (physical sensations), cognitive (the ways people think about their situation), and behavioral (what people do about their situation).

The most common physical feelings of generalized anxiety include gastrointestinal and stomach issues, including nausea, vomiting, and diarrhea. Many people with anxiety end up with ulcers. Other common issues include frequent headaches and bruxism (clenching or grinding of the teeth).

Cognitive reactions to stress—the way you think about anxiety—may make it worse. For instance, if someone is constantly worrying about getting sick to their stomach, they may actually bring on the sickness. Someone with GAD may also become very sensitive emotionally, feeling criticized, edgy, irritable, or jittery.

Behavior can also worsen the symptoms of anxiety. Avoiding certain situations will reinforce the fears already associated with that situation. Why? When you run away from a fearful situation, you likely feel relief. But each time you avoid the stressful event, you're actually strengthening your belief that you're unable to deal successfully with the situation. The temporary reduction of anxiety may feel good, but ultimately it will make overcoming the anxiety far more difficult.

Only a trained professional, such as a psychologist, social worker, outpatient therapist, psychiatrist, or clinical nurse, can make a proper diagnosis of an anxiety disorder. If these symptoms sound familiar, reach out to a trusted adult to find help.

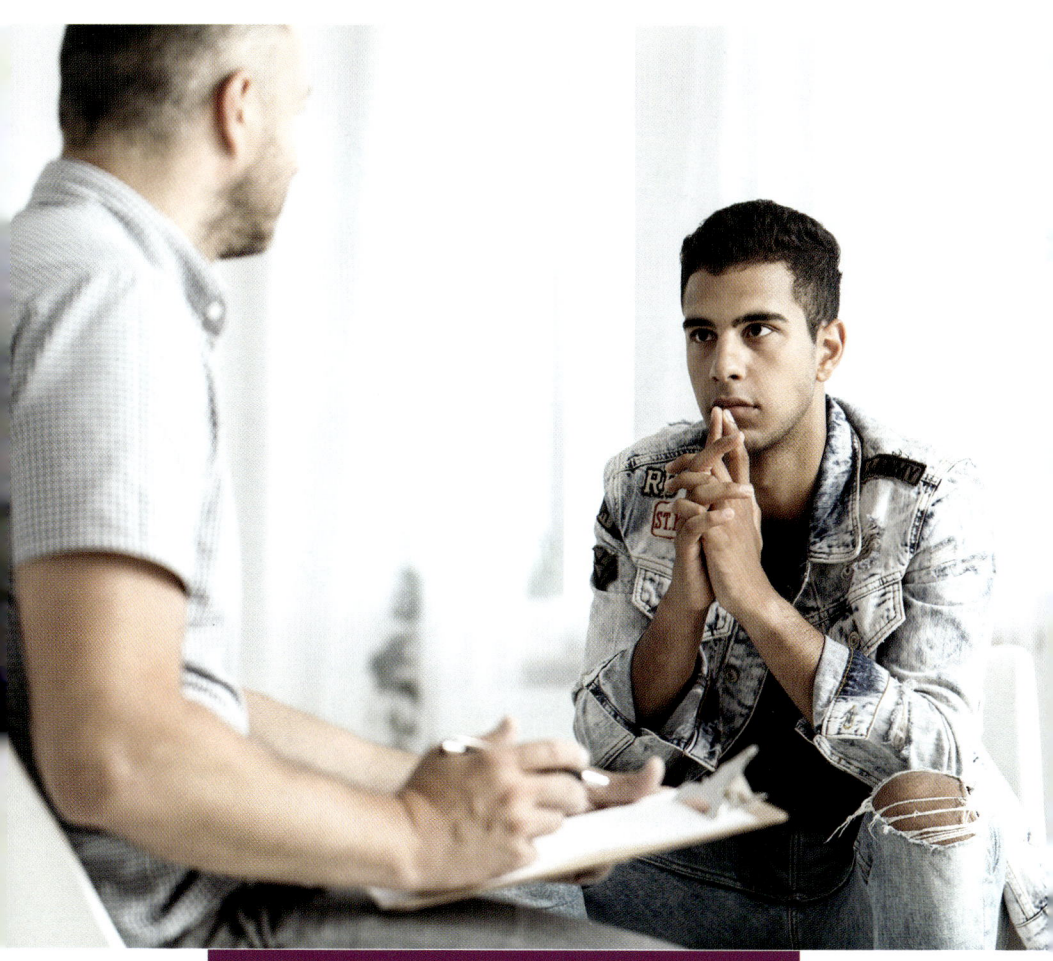

You might be very worried about reaching out to someone to find help for your anxiety, but it can make all the difference.

PTSD

As discussed earlier, while panic disorder is characterized by panic attacks with no obvious reason, other anxiety disorders can also result in panic

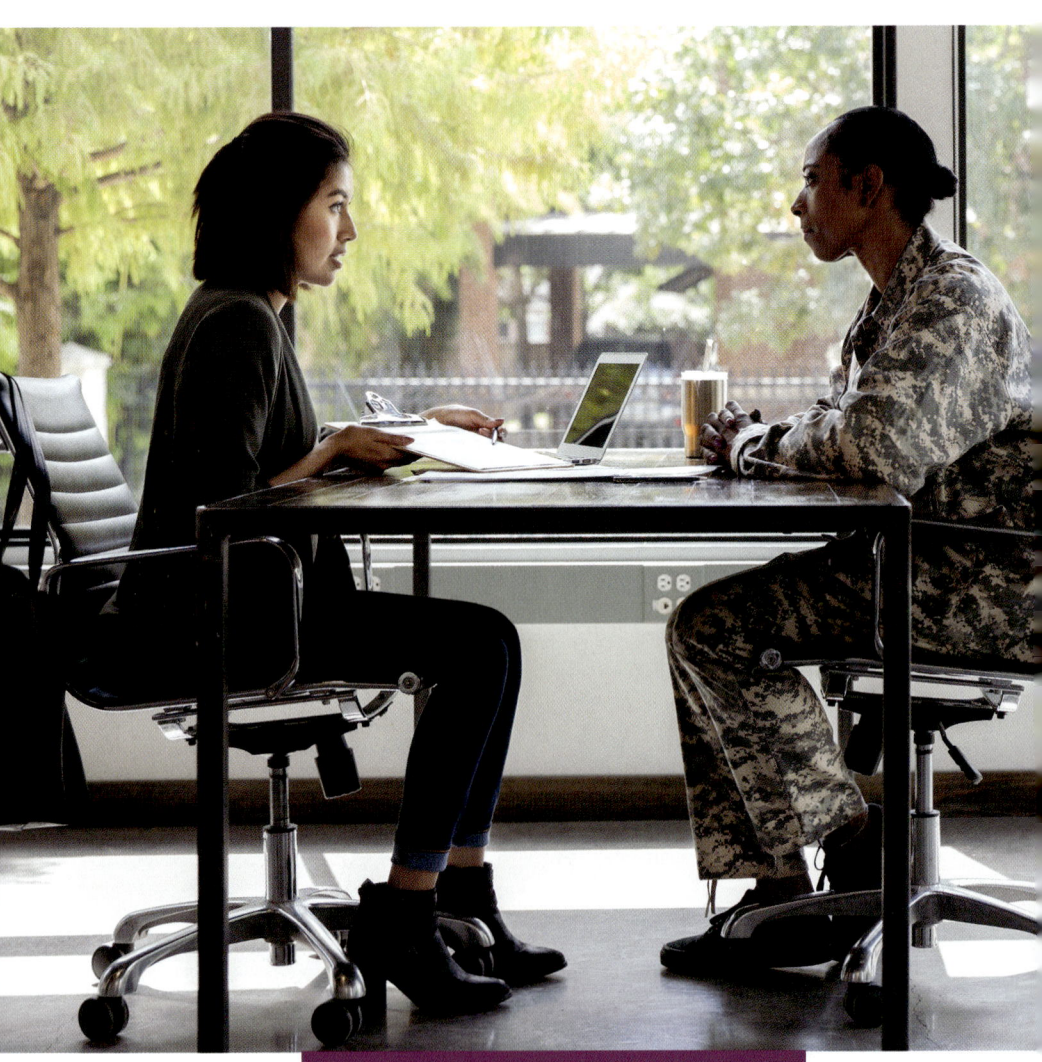

Veterans often have to deal with PTSD. However, anyone who's been through trauma may develop it.

attacks. People who deal with post-traumatic stress disorder may have panic attacks when confronted with reminders of trauma. People who have been abused or who have witnessed or experienced natural disasters (such as tornadoes, fires, and floods) or man-made disasters (such as shootings, car accidents, and kidnappings), have all been through traumas.

People who suffer from PTSD show three major symptoms: hypervigilance (being on guard at all times), intrusion (thinking about the trauma, having nightmares), and constriction (limiting their lifestyle to avoid thinking about the trauma). The hypervigilance and intrusion lead to panic attacks, and the constriction may lead to agoraphobia as the person tries to avoid situations reminiscent of the trauma.

SOCIAL PHOBIAS

When people start to avoid certain situations, they're often on their way to developing phobias. Social phobias feature a fear of embarrassing oneself in public. Social phobias are very common among teenagers. The most common social phobia is the fear of speaking in public, followed by the fear of choking.

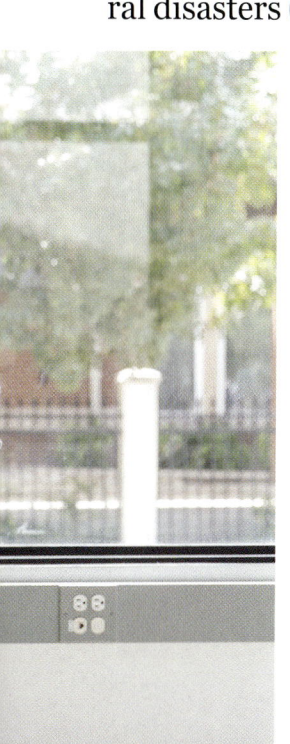

Although social phobias frequently begin in late childhood and extend into a person's early 20s, most people seem to outgrow them. Social phobias differ from simple phobias in that the real fear is of embarrassing yourself. People may be afraid of using the bathroom, eating, using the telephone, or even signing their name in public. People who suffer from social phobias typically fear being observed, thinking that others are laughing at them or finding fault with them. As a result, they start avoiding places where they may feel these things are happening.

How can you tell if a person has agoraphobia or a social phobia? If the person avoids going to the mall or the grocery store out of fear of doing something embarrassing, the person has a social phobia. If the person avoids going to those same places because he or she is afraid of having a panic attack, he or she suffers from agoraphobia.

Some people who have panic attacks develop phobias. They experience a panic attack and then try to find a logical explanation for it. If they panicked while driving down the highway, they associate the panic attack with the highway. Then they avoid driving on the highway. The avoidance reinforces the fear and contributes to the development of a phobia. Since avoidance brings relief, people are encouraged to run away from their fear. By running away, they are telling themselves that the fearful situation is too overwhelming for them to handle. As a result, the phobia grows.

OCD

As briefly discussed early, obsessive-compulsive disorder means having persistent, distressing thoughts and repeating either certain behaviors (like hand washing or checking) or mental acts (like praying or counting) to cancel out these thoughts.

OCD has two distinct parts: obsessions and compulsions. Obsessions are thoughts that won't go away. They are unwanted, uncontrollable, and often inappropriate thoughts, such as thinking you might stab someone with a knife that's lying on the kitchen counter. Compulsions then develop in response to obsessions. Repeating certain physical or mental tasks over and over helps to buy some relief from the anxiety of the obsession.

Everyone has inappropriate thoughts from time to time, and everyone has routines, but someone is said to have obsessive-compulsive disorder when a routine interferes with the rest of his or her life.

The most common compulsion is checking. Some people check to see if they have turned off the stove, turned out the lights, or locked the front door. They don't just check once or twice; they may check 20 or 30 times. Other people have compulsions to touch things, certain rituals for walking through doorways, or certain ways of getting dressed for school or work each day. Failing to perform their rituals brings them excruciating discomfort.

| 42 | I GET PANIC ATTACKS...WHAT'S NEXT? |

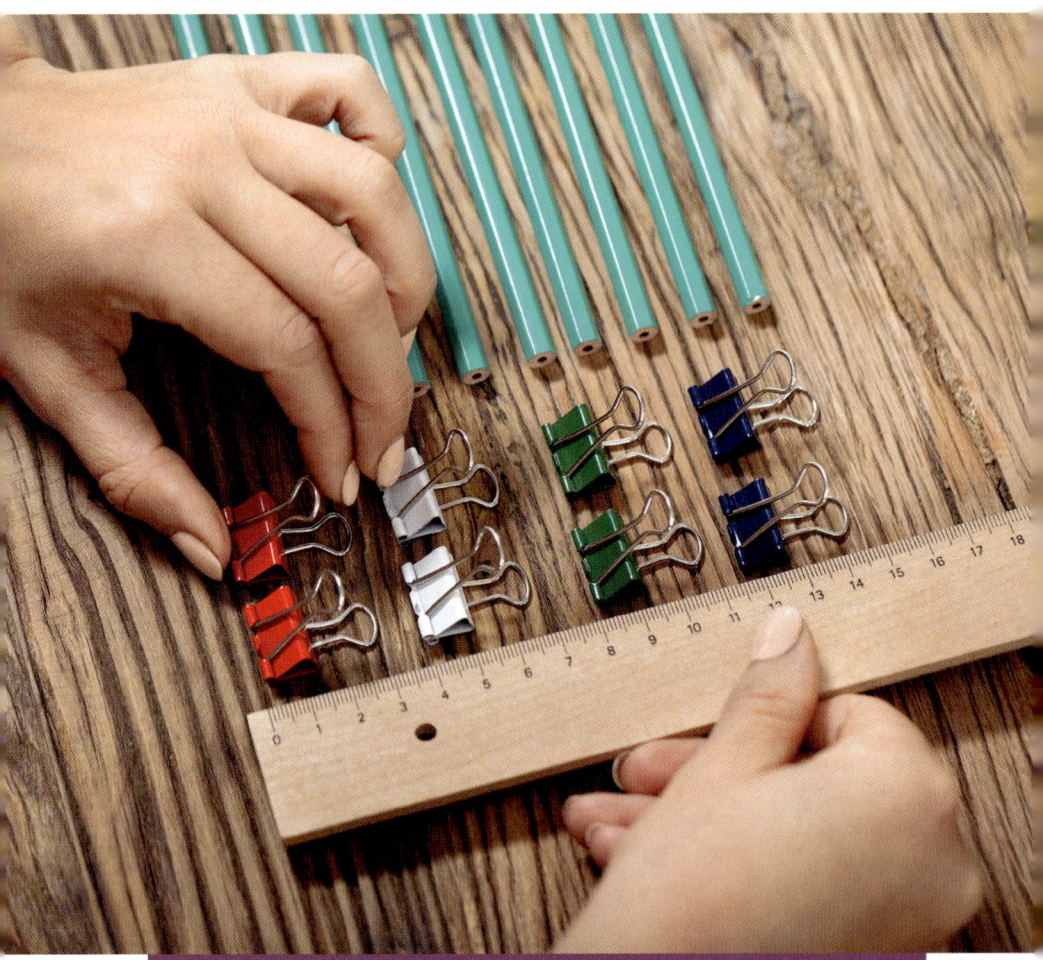

Some people like to joke that they have OCD when they just like things a particular way. True OCD is far more serious. It can seriously affect a person's life.

The reasoning, which is sometimes called magical thinking, goes like this: "If I perform this ritual right or say something five times in a row, nothing bad will happen to me (or to a loved one)." The fear that something bad will happen drives the person with OCD to perform rituals over and over until they "feel" that they have been done correctly.

The rituals or litanies (spoken phrases) are usually connected to the obsessive worries in some way. Someone who constantly fears doing something blasphemous (antireligious) may pray compulsively; someone who is obsessed with contamination may compulsively wash his or her hands. In some cases, the connection between the obsessions and the compulsions may not be obvious or logical to anyone other than the person with OCD.

THE LINK TO DEPRESSION

It's very common for someone with an anxiety disorder to have experienced depression. In fact, about half of those diagnosed with one also have the other. Anxiety can be a symptom of major depression, and an anxiety disorder can be a trigger for depression.

Depression is more than just feeling sad. It's a serious disorder that requires treatment. Symptoms include feelings of despair and hopelessness, loss of energy or concentration, lack of interest in life or activities, changes in sleep, appetite, or movement, and suicidal thoughts. It doesn't have a single cause but can often be traced back to the same things that may cause anxiety.

More than 19 million adults in the United States have likely had a depressive episode in the past year. Depression tends to affect more women than men. More than 264 million people worldwide live with depression, including many teenagers.

Depression can look somewhat different in teens than in older people. Irritability and anger may be

(continued on the next page)

I GET PANIC ATTACKS...WHAT'S NEXT?

(continued from the previous page)

more common symptoms than sadness. You may have unexplained aches and pains, such as stomachaches. You might feel worthless, especially if you often tend to be an overachiever. You may want to withdraw from some of your friends or family members.

However, depression can be treated, especially if it's diagnosed quickly. If you think you might be clinically depressed (or you think a friend might be), talk to a trusted adult. And if you or a friend are having suicidal thoughts, you can call the National Suicide Prevention Lifeline at 1-800-273-TALK.

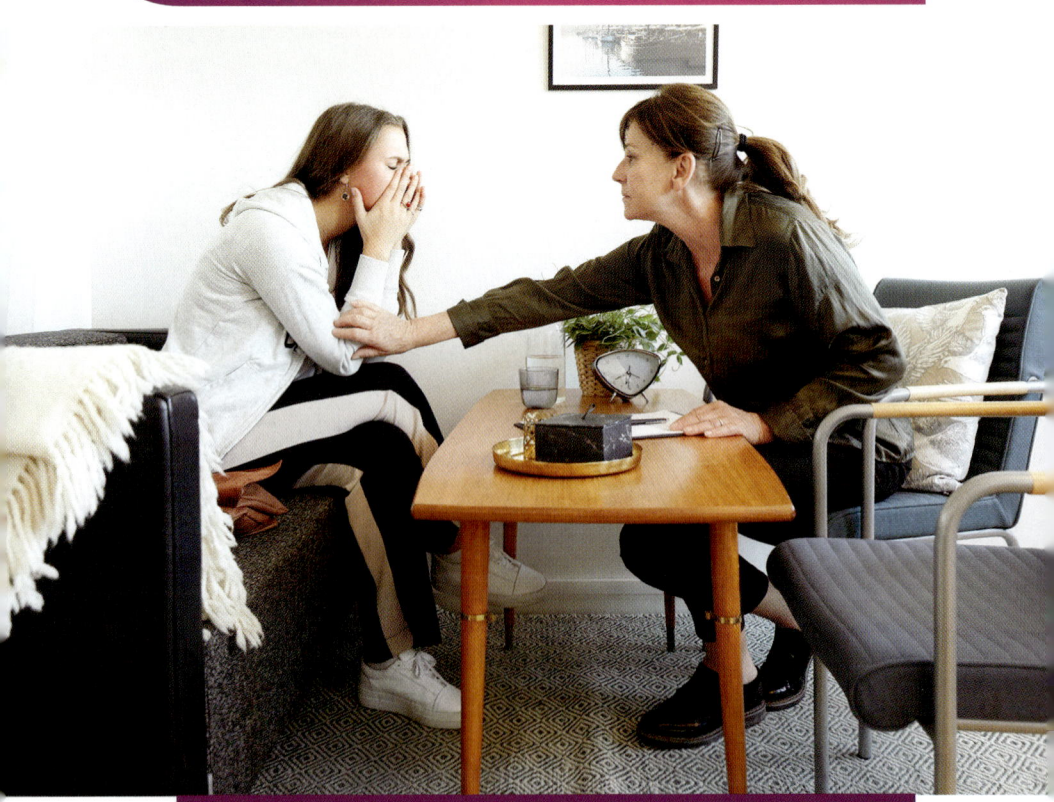

There may seem to be no way out of major depression, but it can be treated. It's important to talk to a trusted adult if you think you might be depressed.

THE SCIENCE OF PANIC ATTACKS

Panic is the body's way of preparing a person to flee or fight when encountering a threat. Fear or panic are normal reactions to danger. They set off a chain of events in the body by activating the autonomic nervous system, which controls breathing, digestion, and temperature regulation.

The autonomic nervous system is composed of two parts: the sympathetic nervous system (SNS) and the parasympathetic nervous system (PNS). The job of the SNS is to rev a person up, whereas the job of the PNS is to calm that person down. The two parts balance each other out. When someone's frightened, the SNS releases adrenaline with dramatic results. Their heart pumps harder to make their blood circulate more quickly through their body to where it's most needed. The person is aware only of their pounding, racing heart or the tingling sensations in their hands and feet. That's because blood is being diverted from the hands and feet to the larger muscles.

The lungs get into the action too. They work harder to draw in more air. The person starts to breathe harder and faster and to sweat. The adrenaline causes them to focus more intently on the immediate danger. Their body is now totally aroused and ready to fight.

Were it not for the PNS, this person's body would remain on high alert indefinitely, and the heightened responses would wreak havoc with their health. Thus, once the danger is past, the PNS takes over, destroying the adrenaline and bringing the body back into a relaxed state.

A panic attack occurs when the body has these heightened responses although no danger is present. The SNS is activated, but since there's no danger to contend with, the body can't get rid of the adrenaline. Eventually, the PNS kicks in and the symptoms diminish. In the meantime, the person may be left wondering if they're about to die. Since they see no visible danger, they decide the danger is inside them. They may think they're having a heart attack.

Many anxious people run to the nearest emergency room only to learn that their EKG reveals no sign of heart trouble. They're told they've had a panic attack. In an attempt to make sense of the panic, they look for a possible cause. Once they think they've located that cause, they avoid it in the future. This avoidance may eventually lead to agoraphobia.

Agoraphobia literally means "a fear of the marketplace," and people often assume that this means a fear of open places. Yet agoraphobics fear more than just open areas. Above all else, agoraphobics are afraid they will suffer a panic attack in public and not be able to get back to safety. As a result, they fear malls, other people's houses, churches, concert halls, schools, and sports arenas—just about every place except the safety of their own home.

People who have panic attacks are afraid of having further attacks. The sensation of being out of control—experiencing a pounding heart, hyperventilating, sweating, and going numb—is so over-

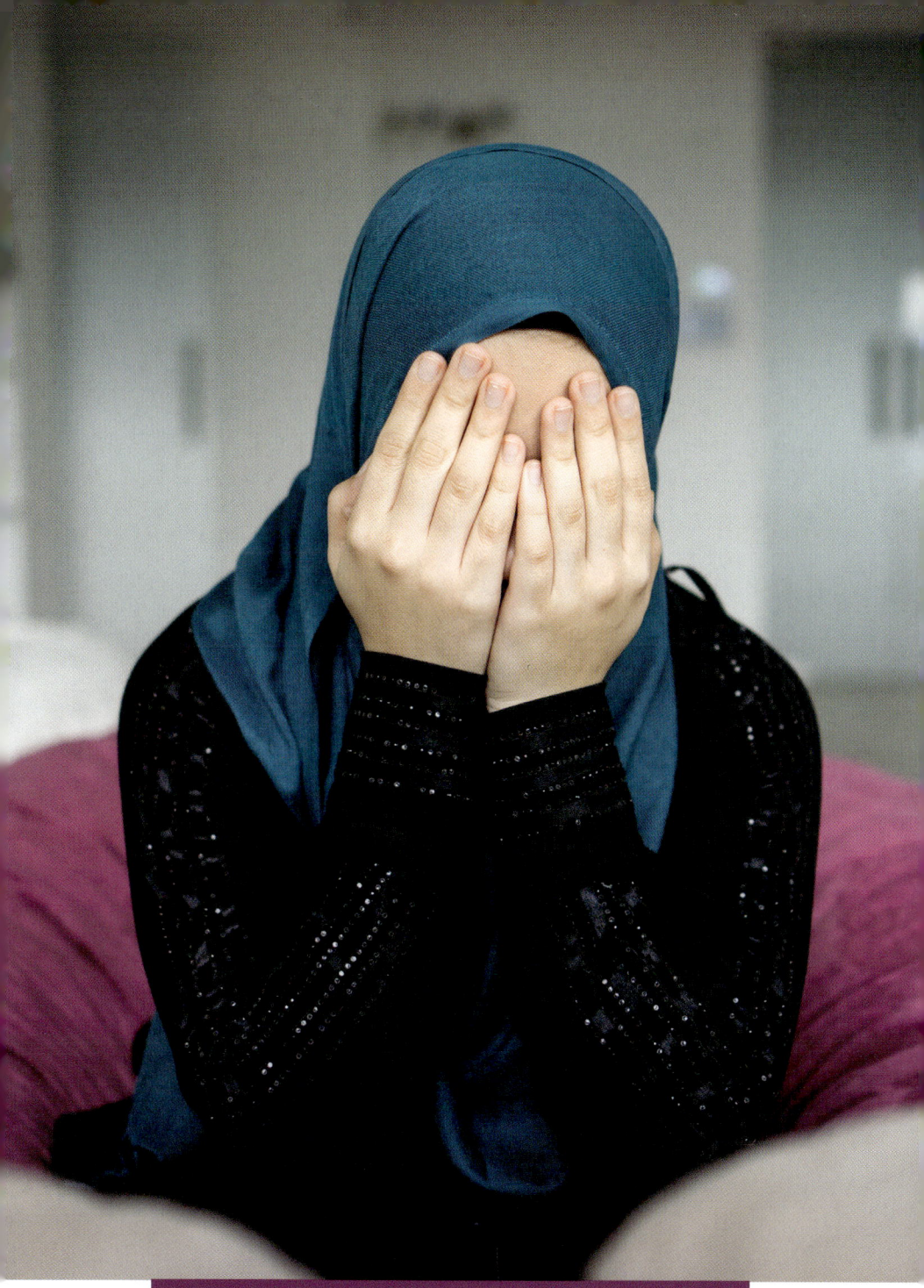

Panic attacks can turn into agoraphobia if people don't deal with them. They want to do anything to keep from having another attack.

whelming that they do almost anything to avoid feeling that way again. For some, it means avoiding any place where escape is difficult. Eventually, people with agoraphobia can't leave the house unless they are with a "safe" person—someone on whom they rely to keep them calm.

Someone who can't leave the safety of his or her home is said to be suffering from panic attacks with agoraphobia. The person who is still willing to go out is said to suffer from panic attacks without agoraphobia.

A WIDE VARIETY

These are only some of the anxiety disorders that exist. There are many types and combinations, and only a professional diagnosis can help someone figure out exactly which ones or combinations they might be experiencing and what other issues (physiological or mental) might be complicating things.

Whatever you're dealing with, however, you're not alone. Many people deal with these anxiety disorders, as well as depression and other mental health issues. Help is out there.

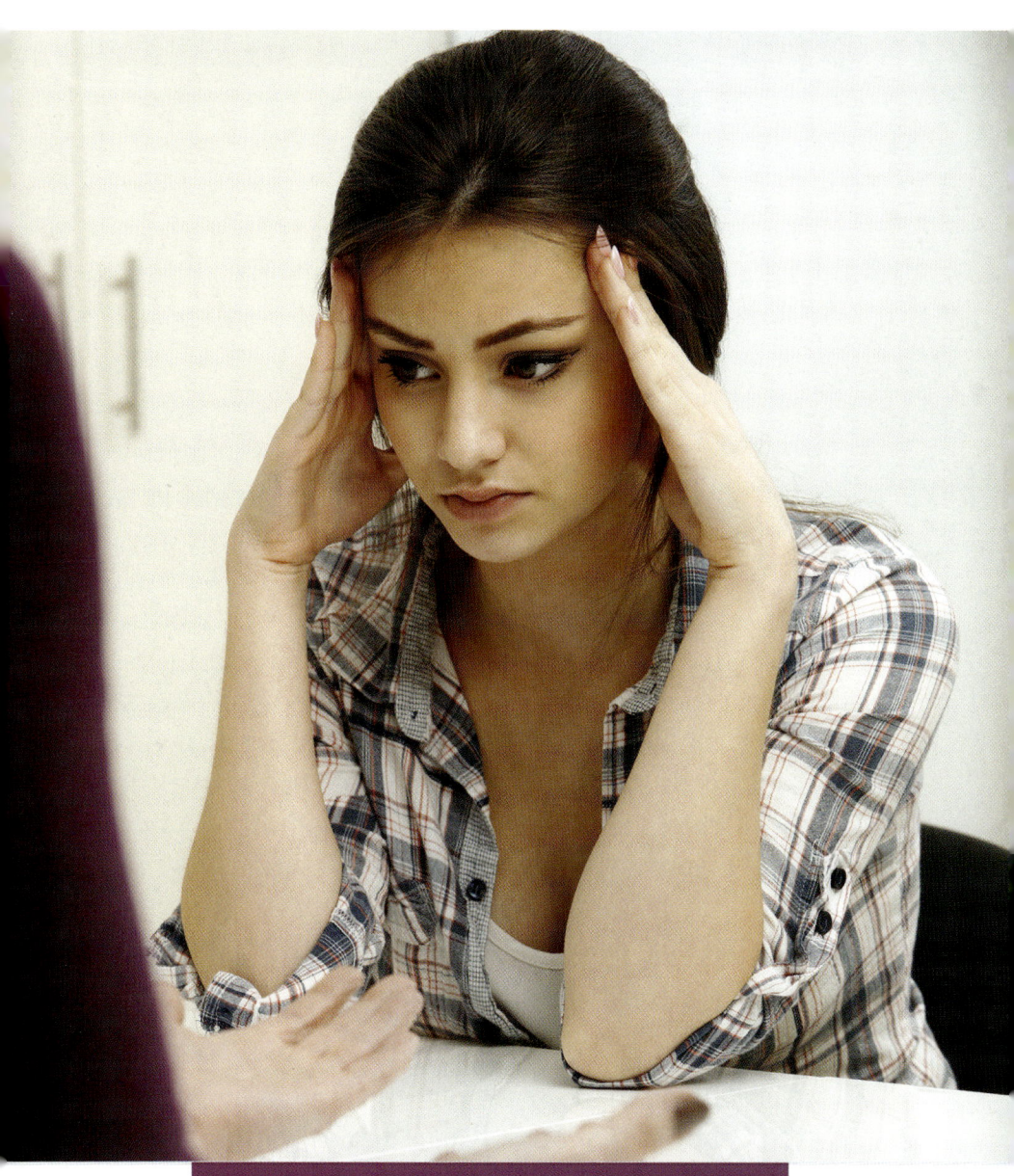

If you're dealing with anxiety and depression, don't give up. It might take a while to find the best way to help you, but help is out there. You can find it. And you don't have to live like this.

CHAPTER 4

WHAT CAN YOU DO?

While anxiety and panic attacks may make you feel helpless, the good news is that there are treatments for these issues. This could include both medication and psychotherapy—often known as talk therapy. The essence of traditional psychotherapy is to bring the original conflict to light, whether by examining defense mechanisms or by talking about feelings. Since people manage their anxiety through unconscious means, it's a therapist's job to expose the person's defense mechanisms. By gaining insight into the source of the anxiety, the person may be better able to manage it. However, psychotherapy alone isn't always enough.

TALK THERAPY

When the field of psychoanalysis began, people often believed that anxiety came from wanting to do something a person knew was not acceptable. This conflict, people thought, could originate in childhood. If a person was unable to face these unacceptable urges, they would divert the urges into specific

WHAT CAN YOU DO?   51

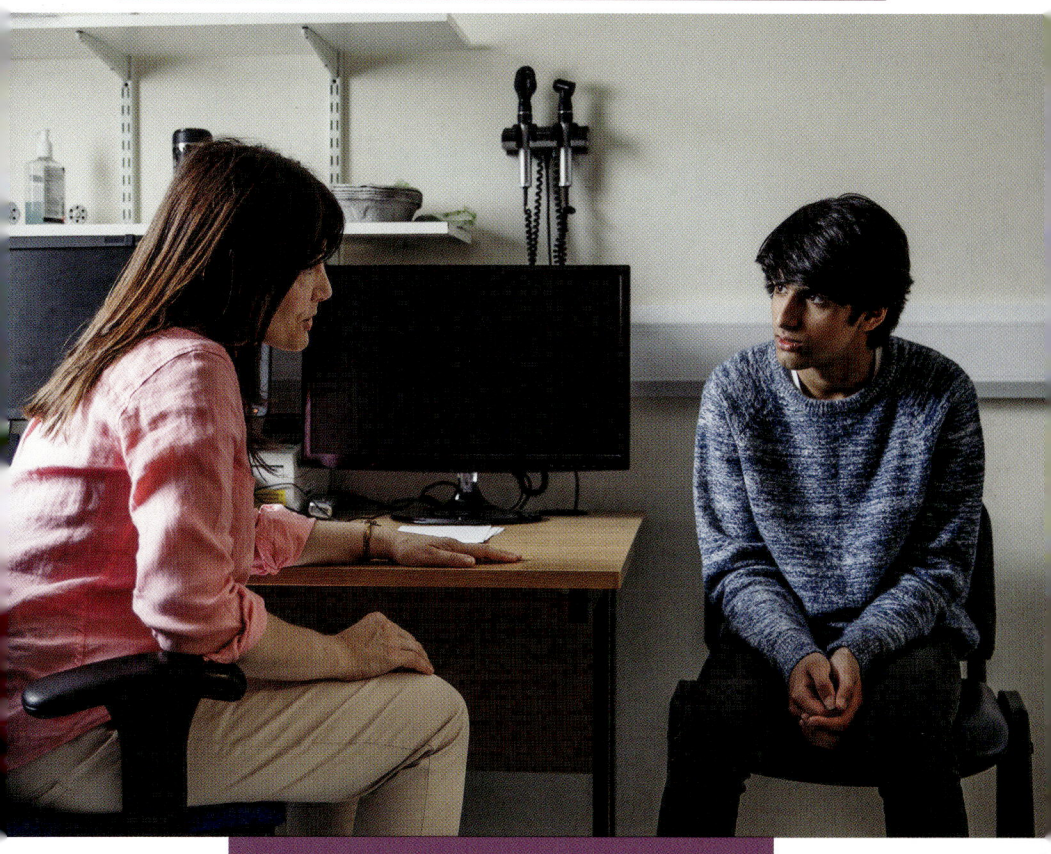

A doctor can help you understand if talk therapy might be right for you and can help you find the right therapist.

phobias or feel compelled to perform certain behaviors over and over.

People developed psychoanalysis to study the origins of anxiety. Modern therapists may also try to connect a person's present conflict with some unresolved conflict in the past. The emphasis is on remembering the original conflict and talking it out. The problem is that often, knowing the source of the anxiety does not necessarily help stop it.

Defense mechanisms can keep people unaware of their anxiety. All defense mechanisms are unconscious; people are not aware of them at the time they use them. A therapist's job is to bring defense mechanisms to their patients' attention so that they understand the source of their anxiety. At that point, people may be able to learn how to deal with the feelings of anxiety. There are many different kinds of defense mechanisms.

REPRESSION

When someone represses certain bad memories, they basically forget them. This doesn't happen intentionally; it just happens, usually when the memories are so horrible that they would cause great anxiety if they were remembered. Of course, repressed memories haven't fully disappeared. They're just removed from someone's awareness, although they still have enormous power to motivate people to behave in certain ways that they can't quite explain.

REGRESSION

A person resorts to regression when they feel overwhelmed by stress; they begin to behave in a way more suited to an earlier, less stressful time. For example, a four-year-old who has a new baby sister may become stressed by all the attention his parents are giving the baby. As a result, they may start to act more babyish.

RATIONALIZATION

If you've ever arrived in class without your homework and blamed it on the parents who sent you to bed early, you know what rationalization is. When someone rationalizes, they come up with a seemingly plausible explanation for their actions. The explanation usually absolves the person from blame, thereby alleviating some of the stress or anxiety about a situation.

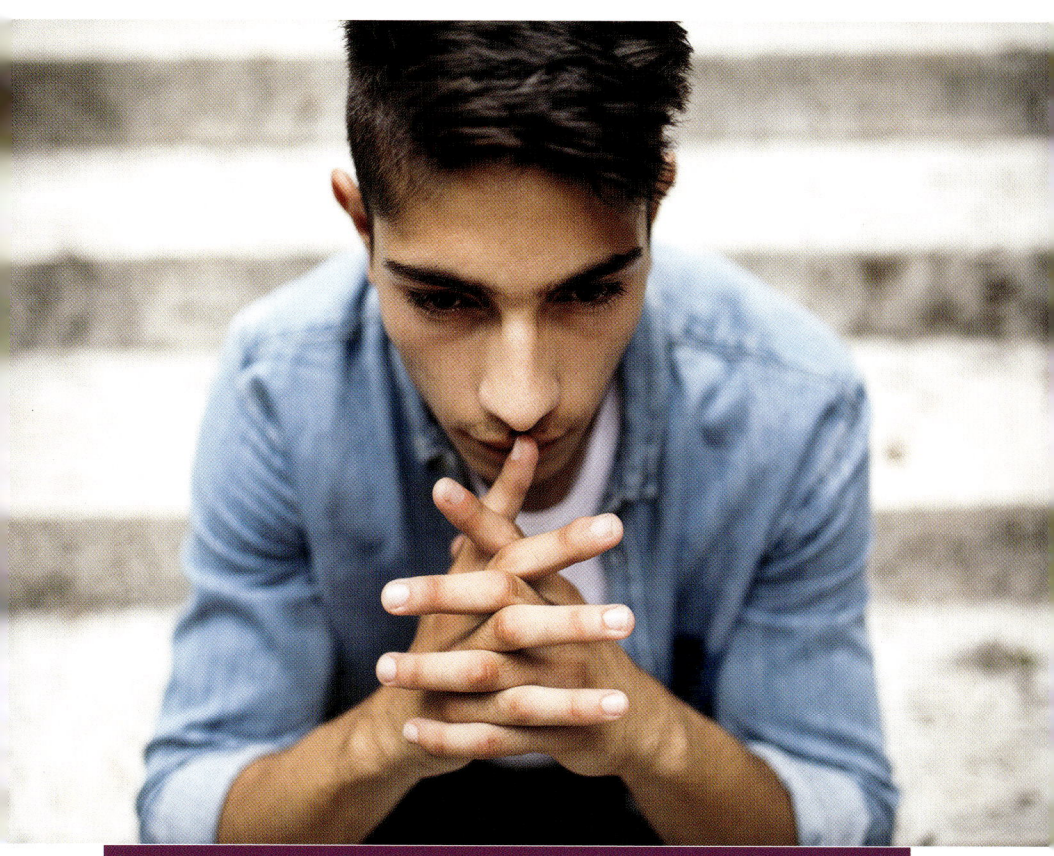

It can be easy to fall into common defense mechanisms. However, this doesn't really help you deal with your anxiety and other issues. You need to face the problems.

DISPLACEMENT

Taking out feelings on someone or something other than the cause of those feelings is called displacement. For example, a student may get angry at their teacher about something and go home and yell at their sister for something unrelated. Really, though, they're angry with the teacher for assigning homework on a night they had plans or something similar. Unable to let out their anger at their teacher, they displace it on to their sister.

PROJECTION

This occurs when someone disowns certain qualities that they don't like about themselves and starts to attribute those qualities to other people. For example, a person who can't accept that they're a gossip may unjustly accuse their friend of gossiping.

REACTION FORMATION

This defense mechanism occurs when a person can't accept their own negative feelings but makes themself believe that their feelings are really the opposite. A young person who hates their father for treating them badly tells themselves that they really adore their father. When other people say bad things about their father, the young person defends him. It's not a case of pretending to like their father. They convince themselves that they really have such positive feelings.

DIFFERENT TYPES OF THERAPIES

Cognitive and behavioral therapies involve more than just talking about anxiety and determining its root conflict. Cognitive therapists focus on changing a person's thinking, and behavioral therapists focus on changing their behavior. Many therapists use both approaches in an attempt to treat the disorder.

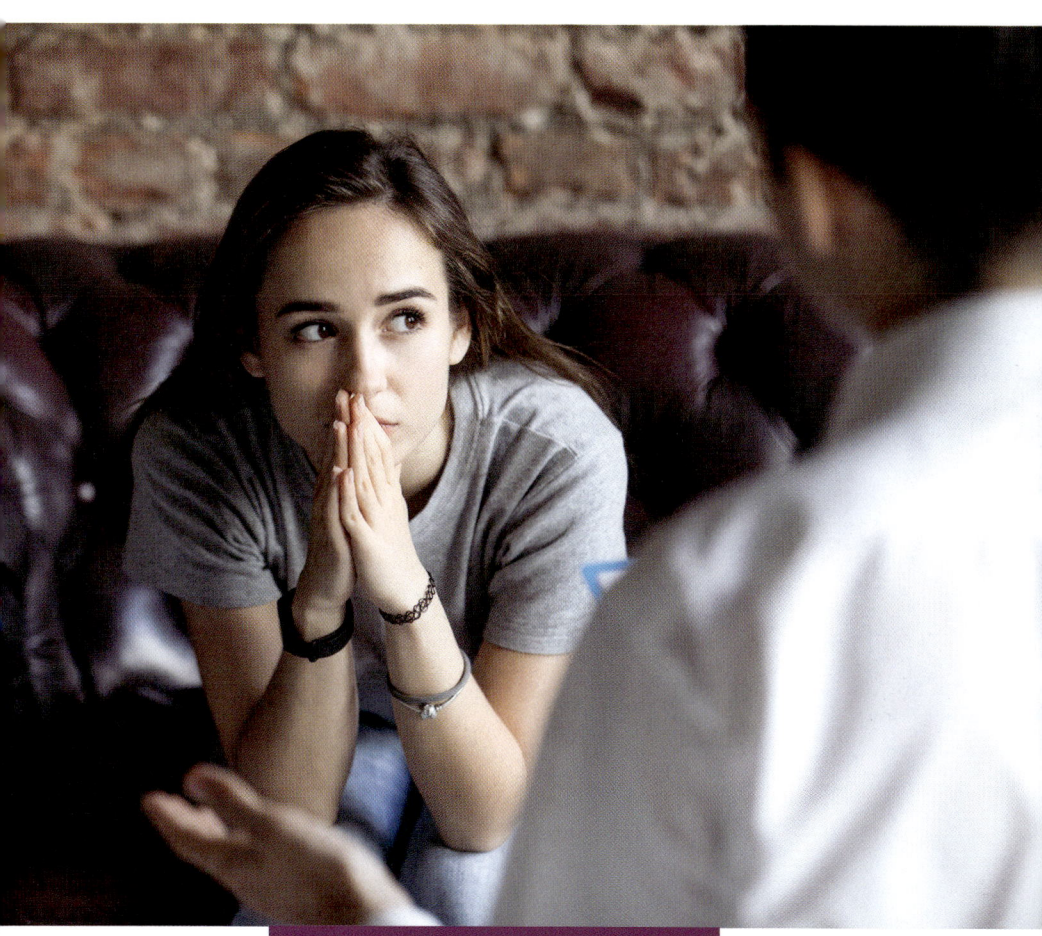

Talking to a therapist can be scary. It might take a while to find one that's perfect for you.

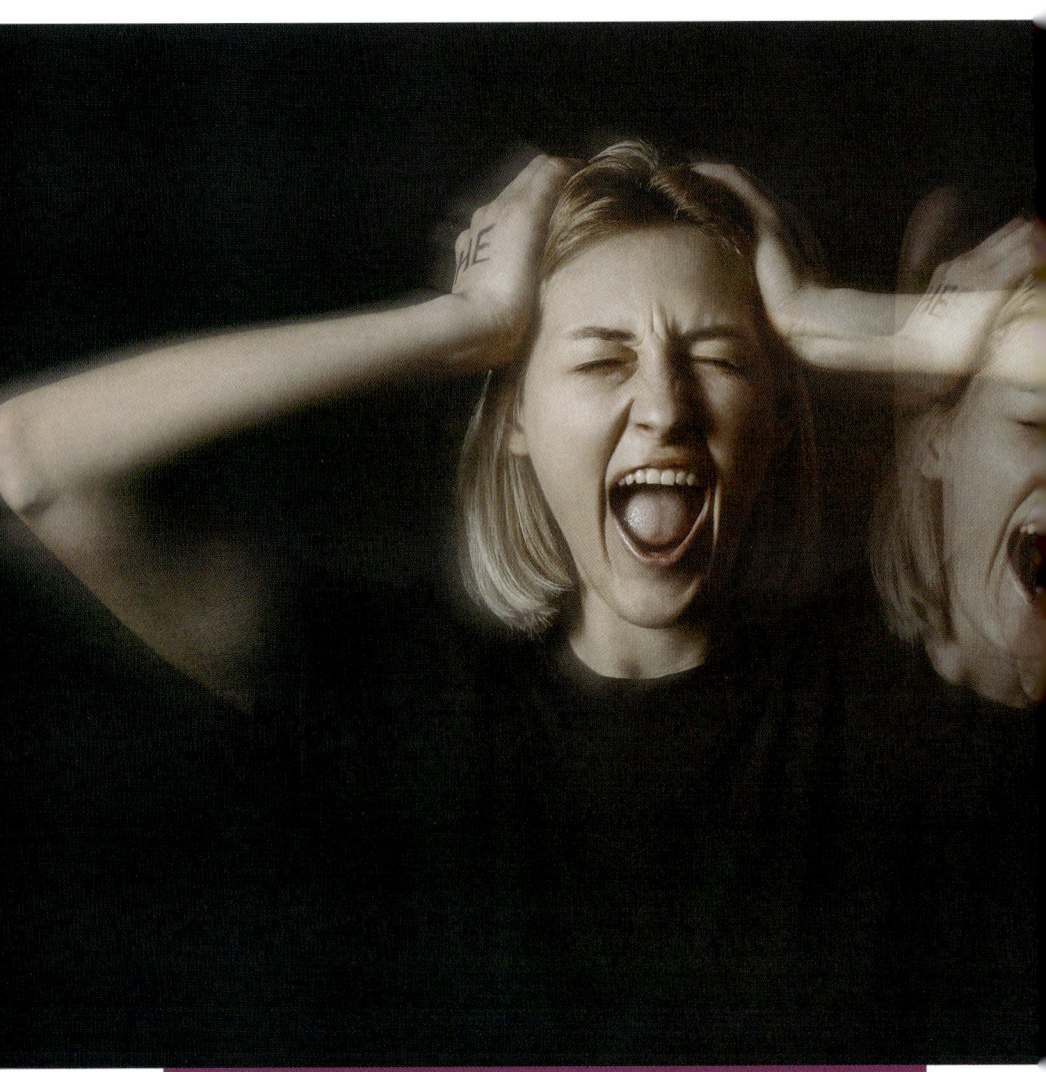

A bad panic attack might make you feel as if the world is ending. It's important not to fall into negative self-talk. That only makes things worse.

Physiological reasons may explain the beginnings of panic and phobias, but what people think and what they do about these conditions determines how well they are able to cope with them.

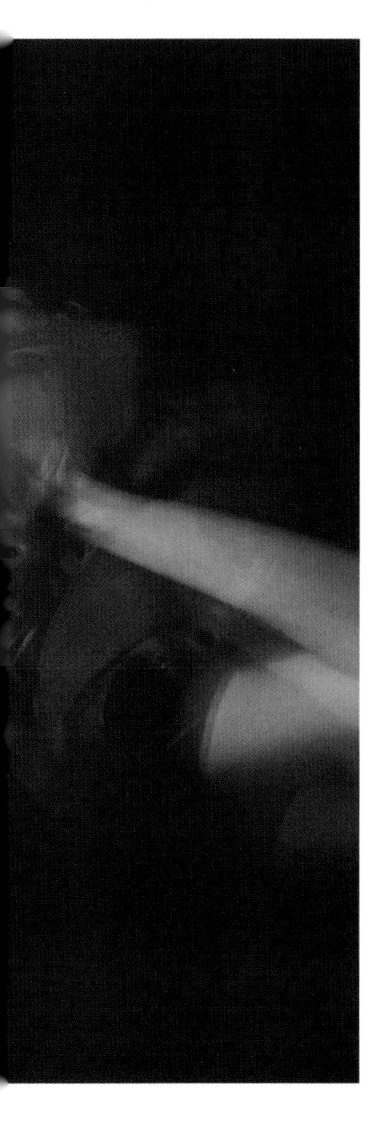

As mentioned earlier, some people worsen their anxiety with negative self-talk. They convince themselves they can't handle it when they feel a panic attack coming on. They start telling themselves that they can't possibly handle a situation and that it will only get worse. Their anxiety escalates.

However, a cognitive therapist may tell someone to change their self-talk and make it positive. They may suggest the person tell themselves that they can handle the situation. If they feel anxious, they think that this happens to everyone. If they have a panic attack, they can tell themselves that they can ride out the symptoms. A panic attack lasts only 10 to 20 minutes at most, and they can tolerate discomfort that long. People can learn to challenge their mistaken beliefs about their situation and their ability to handle it.

Earlier, it was mentioned how people can think negatively in ways that include overgeneralizing, all-or-nothing thinking, exaggeration, catastrophic thinking (or catastrophizing), and underestimating themselves. Most of the time people make these types of statements to themselves without stopping to challenge the truth of them. If you want to reduce your anxiety, you must first learn to recognize your mistaken beliefs. Then you have to look for what's wrong about that belief and challenge it, substituting more supportive thoughts. Cognitive therapists understand that it isn't so much the event that leads to anxiety as it is the way someone feels about the event.

Making up a list can help people become more aware of their own mistaken beliefs. This list could include the following:

- The event
- Their thoughts about the event
- Cognitive distortion in that thinking
- Ways to challenge negative self-talk by substituting more supportive thoughts

The purpose of refraining from negative self-talk is to keep anxiety from escalating. When something happens or someone anticipates a scary event, their negative self-talk could lead them to feel anxious. If they look at the mistaken beliefs in their thinking and challenge them with more realistic, affirming statements, their anxiety should decrease. After all, it's not the event that makes them anxious; it's how they think about the event.

CATASTROPHE!

Catastrophic thinking isn't unusual in people who deal with anxiety disorders. In fact, it's common in kids and teenagers. People who are prone to this are constantly scanning their world and their future, looking ahead to disasters and worst-case scenarios. A teen who tends to do this may convince themselves that if they fail one test, they'll never get into college or that the lack of an invitation to one party means that everyone at school hates them.

This kind of thinking can make depression and anxiety far worse. It can lead people to avoid situations, people, and places. It's usually not intentional; people do it without realizing it. Fatigue can make catastrophic thinking much worse.

If you tend to fall prey to catastrophic thinking, one way to deal with it is to face the thought, no matter how hard it is. You weren't invited to a party. What if everyone at school hates you? Then, you examine the thought. Perhaps you realistically know that's not true, because you were hanging out with a group of good friends just that day. Are they really so good at pretending that you couldn't tell if they didn't like you? Unlikely! However, no one is ever going to be liked by everyone—and maybe the person hosting this one party isn't someone you know well. Finally, you can replace the catastrophic thought with a more realistic scenario. The person hosting the party doesn't know you yet. Maybe when they do, you'll be invited to their parties. Even if they don't invite you, you still have friends. It's not always easy to do this, but it can help.

WAYS TO COPE WITH PANIC

Before someone can learn to tolerate a panic attack or manage the anxiety associated with a phobia, they have to learn how to relax. If they practice it consistently, they will be aware when their muscles are tense and will know how to shake them loose.

When a person breathes properly, their abdomen, not their chest, should rise and fall. Chest breathing is too shallow and doesn't help you relax. To make sure you are breathing correctly, you can lie on your back in a relaxed position. Place one hand on your belly and the other on your chest. Inhale slowly. The hand resting on your belly should rise more than the hand resting on your chest.

If that isn't the case, practice exaggerating the movements as you inhale and exhale. Push your belly out as you inhale and deflate it when you exhale. Concentrate as much on exhaling as you do on inhaling. Not exhaling completely leads to a buildup of carbon dioxide and can lead to feelings of panic.

Then, stand up and continue to breathe, pushing out your abdomen. By exhaling completely, you'll be forced to breathe more slowly and deeply. To ensure that you are breathing slowly at first, inhale to a silent count of 1-2-3. Hold that breath for two counts, then exhale just as slowly to another silent count of 3-2-1. Make sure to breathe through your nose. When you breathe through your mouth, you have a natural tendency to breathe more shallowly.

Now that you know how to relax and breathe properly, you can incorporate these techniques when

WHAT CAN YOU DO? 61

you start to feel anxious. Imagine a ladder with rungs that represent how anxious you are. Mild anxiety is on the bottom rung, progressing up through moderate anxiety to panic at the top.

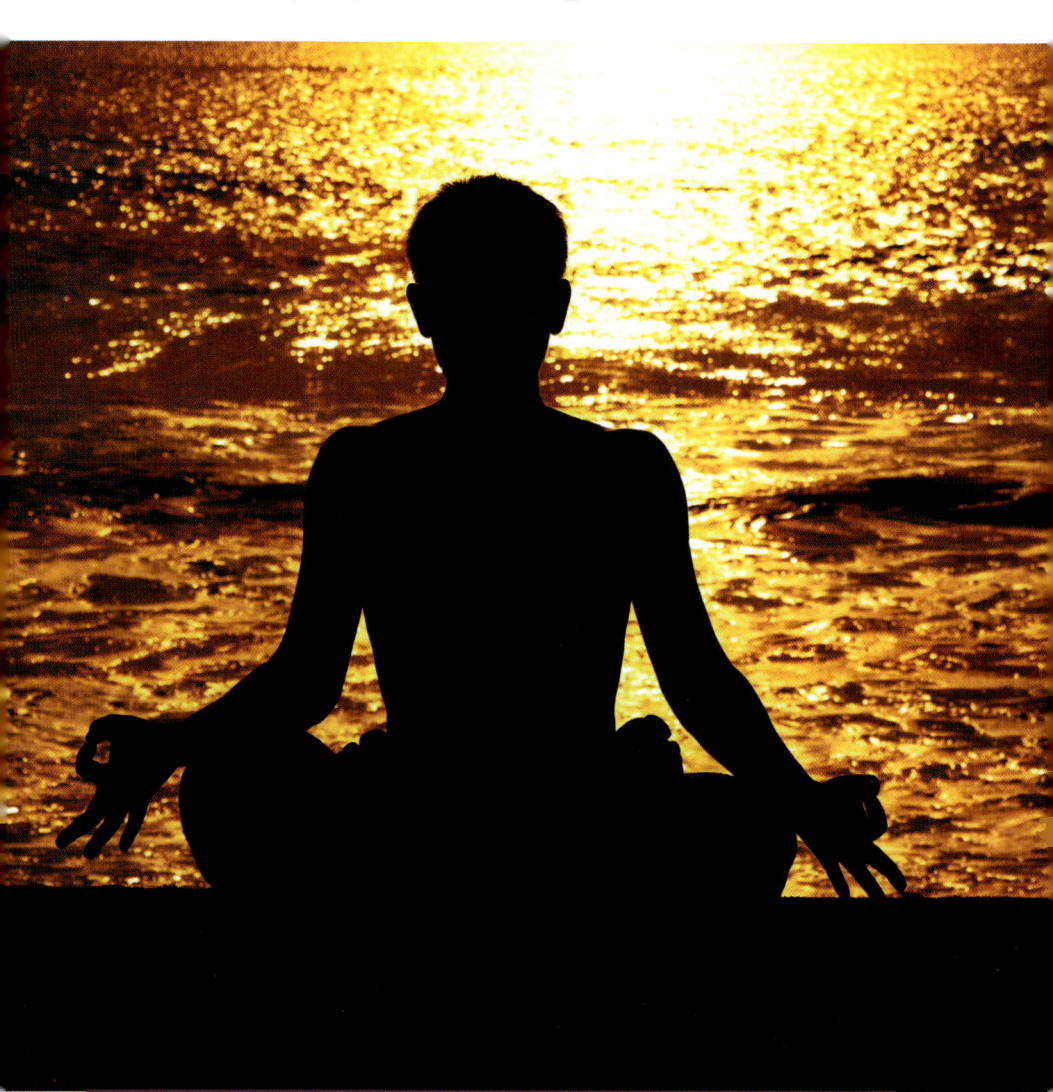

Meditation may be able to help you deal with anxiety. There are many different kinds.

When you are in situations that make you feel anxious, visualize that ladder and where your anxiety fits. If you register only mild anxiety, stay as you are. If you register moderate anxiety, check your body for muscle tension. Relax your muscles and breathe more slowly.

If you find yourself hyperventilating (breathing quickly and in shallow breaths), you can do two things. Try to slow your breathing, which will be the opposite of what your body wants to do. Hold your breath as long as you can, then resume breathing more slowly. Concentrate on exhaling as much as inhaling. If all else fails, breathe into a paper bag (never a plastic bag). Breathing in air you have exhaled can adjust the level of carbon dioxide in your body, helping to calm you down.

DEALING WITH PHOBIAS

The first part of learning to overcome a phobia is getting used to the physical feelings that occur when you're confronted with that phobia. You can learn to get used to them. When you first notice that you're feeling anxious, try to objectively note the sensations. For example, if your heart starts to beat faster, instead of

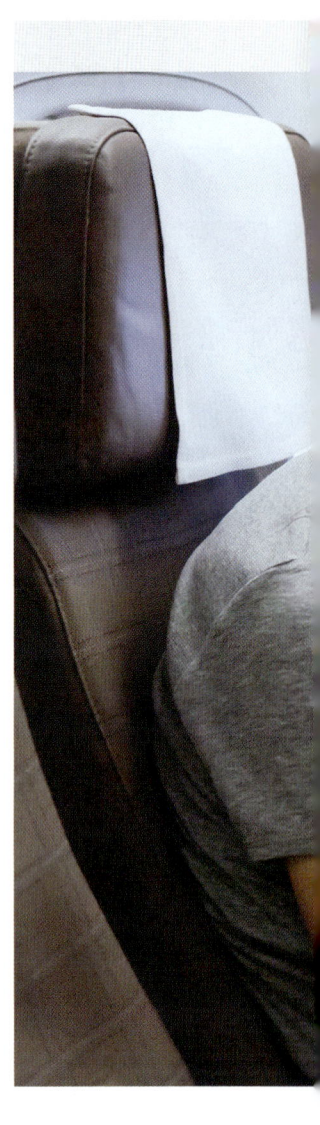

WHAT CAN YOU DO? 63

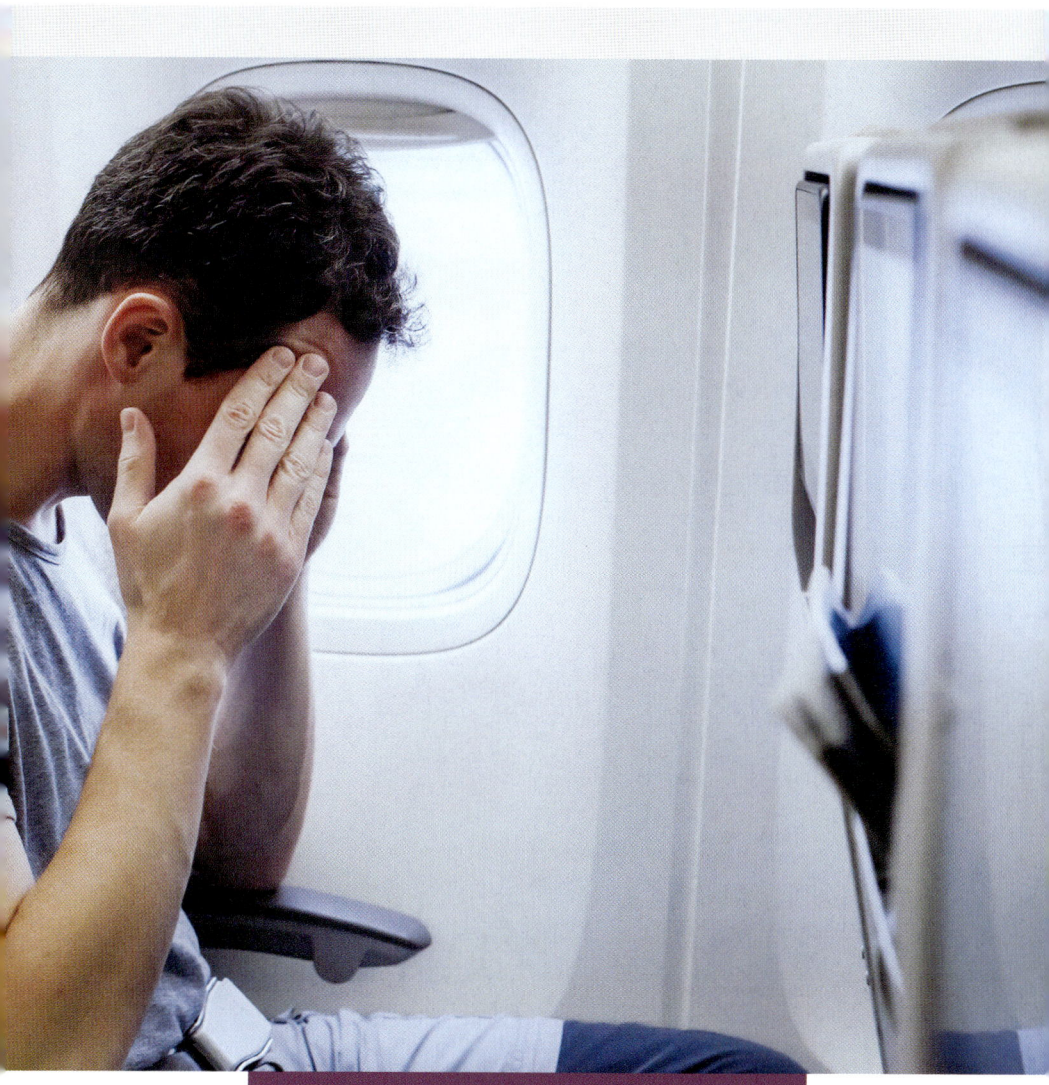

A fear of flying can trigger panic attacks in some people. Learning how to manage your breathing can help.

giving in to panic, simply notice the rapid beating. If your fingers start to feel tingly, wiggle them around and remind yourself that your fingers feel this way

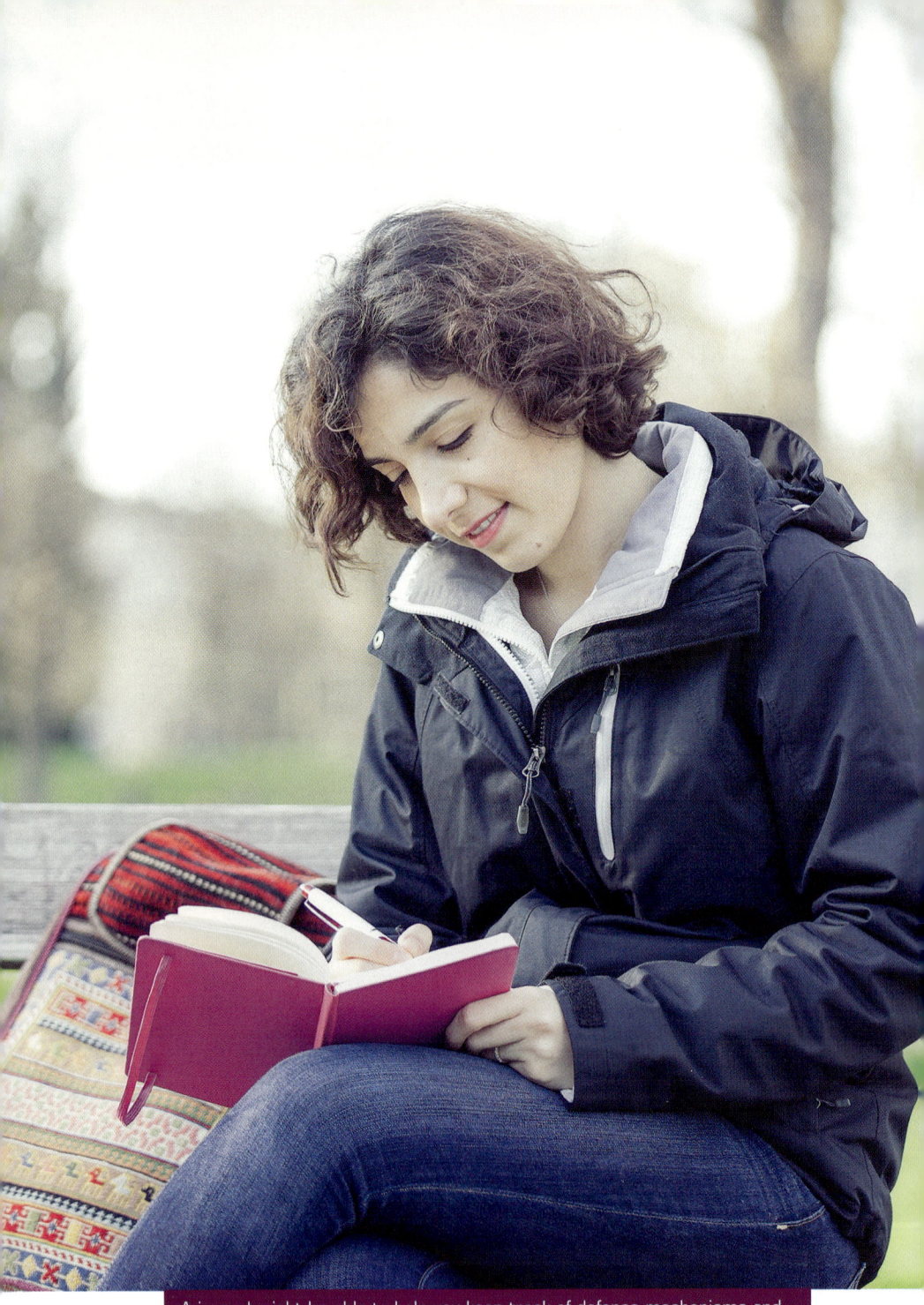

A journal might be able to help you keep track of defense mechanisms and how you can help yourself work through a panic attack. Write down what works for you and what doesn't. It could help you think of these things later.

because an alarm has been triggered in your body and blood is being diverted from your fingertips to your larger muscles.

It may help to write down on a separate sheet of paper all the physical sensations you have. If you're prone to negative thoughts, note what thoughts first come to mind when you sense distress. Challenge the things that aren't true and continue to observe your reactions.

If at any point you feel yourself tensing up, concentrate on relaxing your muscles and breathing more slowly. Continue to observe the feelings as they peak and then subside. Try to remain objective and do not react to the sensations. As they fade, consider which feelings were the most difficult for you. Why these feelings in particular?

As you adjust to uncomfortable feelings, keep using relaxation techniques whenever you catch yourself tensing up. Gradually you may be able to tolerate more and more. Then you're ready for the next step.

Since avoidance of a trigger may only strengthen the phobia, a person with a phobia must face the thing they fear in order to overcome their fear of it. There are a few ways to accomplish this. One is to create a hierarchy of stressful situations, much like the ladder mentioned earlier. At the bottom, list the least stressful of the scenarios. The stress intensifies as you go up the ladder. This is called systematic desensitization. A therapist who specializes in this can help you. Here's how it might go.

A person who's afraid of spiders might envision their hierarchy like this:

SPIDER HIERARCHY

1. Holding a spider in their hand
2. Sitting next to a spider
3. Sitting next to a spiderweb
4. Stepping on a small spider
5. Hearing someone say that a spider ran into their closet
6. Hearing someone say there's a spider in the next room
7. Looking at a spider through a glass barrier in a zoo
8. Looking at a picture of a spider in a magazine

Clearly, just looking at a spider in a magazine is the least stressful scenario, so that's where a person with a spider phobia may begin to desensitize themselves to the fear. If they're a good visualizer, they may start to feel anxious. At that point, they can observe the anxiety and relax their tense muscles. They can take several calming breaths until they can think about the picture without discomfort.

Then they move to the next level, imagining themselves looking at a live spider through a glass barrier at the zoo. As that thought stirs up anxiety, they again need to relax their muscles and take calming breaths. If they're still anxious, they can visualize another scene that calms them. Some people visualize the ocean. Whatever scenario represents a safe, calming place could work.

When the person is calm and relaxed from visualizing their safe place, they can switch back to visualizing the spider. They stay with that scenario until they can visualize it without feeling anxious. They continue up the ladder, visualizing, feeling anxious, and teaching themselves to relax.

Obviously, this is a long process. It's not completed in one sitting or even in one day. By the time this person can imagine holding a spider in her hand without feeling even a twinge of anxiety, they're ready to test themselves by dealing with the real situation.

Exposure involves actually experiencing the anxiety-provoking situations. A phobic person can attempt this either on their own or with their therapist. Clearly, actual exposure is much more anxiety provoking than imagery exposure. It won't be as easy for someone to calm themselves, so they must learn to retreat and recover. When the anxiety has lessened, they can reexpose themselves to the situation and try to increase the time they spend in it. Even if they have to retreat multiple times, they still must reexpose themselves until they can deal with the situation.

When they can tolerate the least stressful situation on the ladder, they move on to the next one, always exposing, calming or retreating, and reexposing. A person with a spider phobia would actually look at a spider in a magazine, not just imagine it. They'd go to the zoo, and they'd actually touch a spider. They would do each of the things on their list until they had conquered their fear of spiders.

WAYS TO DEAL WITH OCD

Obsessive-compulsive disorder is often best treated with medication. However, people sometimes use behavioral techniques in addition to medication. The most successful techniques with obsessive-compulsive disorder are to delay responding to OCD urges and to distract oneself from the anxiety.

A compulsive shopper, for example, would tell themselves to wait until the next day to give in to the shopping urge. Compulsive checkers would tell themselves to wait an hour before getting up to check someone instead of trying to resist the urge entirely. The more they can delay, the more they get used to a little anxiety. Just as someone learns to tolerate discomfort in a panic attack, a person can learn to tolerate the discomfort of ignoring a compulsion.

Reality testing (thinking about what most people would do in the situation and what would really happen) may help someone with OCD learn to dismiss their thoughts without giving in to a compulsion. The goal is to use reality testing to talk themselves into performing fewer compulsions. As they reduce compulsive behavior, they can note their anxiety level. It will be high at first when they choose not to perform a ritual, but when the consequences they're expecting don't actually happen, their anxiety level should go down. Eventually, they may be able to ignore the need to perform certain rituals.

COPING WITH SETBACKS

It's important to realize that setbacks happen. There will be days when you can manage your anxiety by using these ways of coping. Other days, they just won't work as well. Things that cause additional stress, such as an illness, event, or bad night's sleep, may complicate things. Anxiety may get ahold of you again for a while. However, setbacks are temporary. Try to stay positive and keep trying.

CHAPTER 5

MEDICATION MIGHT HELP

Medication can help with panic attacks and anxiety, but it can be a tricky thing. There are a variety of causes for anxiety, and someone may feel anxious because of certain medical conditions or because they have taken prescription or street drugs. The first plan of attack in treating anxiety should be to see a doctor who can rule out any contributing medical problems. Be sure to tell the doctor about all the medicines you've been taking, including any illegal drugs. Your doctor needs to know all the facts. Obviously, if a medical condition is causing the symptoms, that has to be treated first. If this is the case, anxiety may fade as the medical condition is treated. If medications or drugs are causing the symptoms, they have to be changed or stopped altogether.

Also, no drug for anxiety fits every type of disorder or every person. You, with guidance from your doctor, may have to try different doses and types to find one that will work. And no drug is a magic pill or cure-all. Even when you find the right one, it will

MEDICATION MIGHT HELP

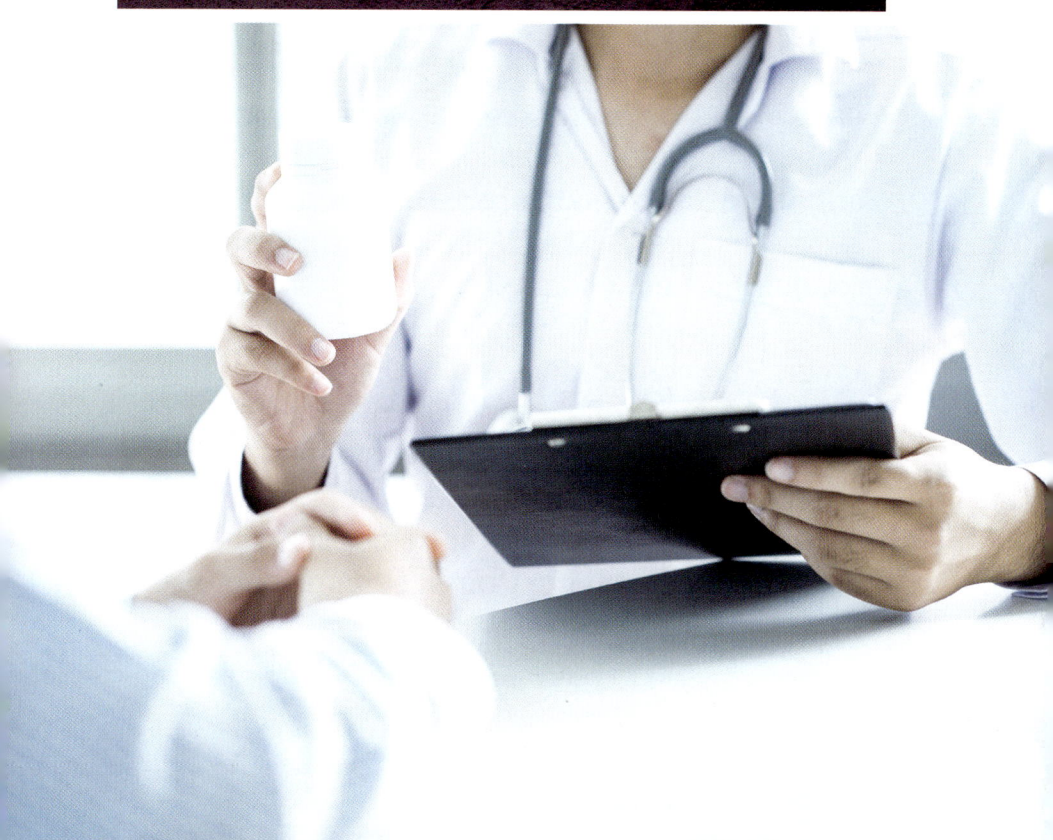

There is no "one size fits all" drug for anxiety. You may have to try a few (with a doctor's oversight) before you find something that helps you.

just assist in managing the symptoms. Still, this can be a big help if you're dealing with anxiety.

KINDS OF MEDICATION

There are a number of types of medication used to treat anxiety disorders. Not all of them are appropriate for teenagers, but your doctor may prescribe a certain kind if they think it will help you.

The most commonly prescribed medicines for panic disorder in teens are selective serotonin reuptake inhibitors (SSRIs). These medications are antidepressants that target the neurotransmitter serotonin and keep the brain's neurons from reabsorbing it too quickly. SSRIs may be prescribed under the names Celexa (citalopram), Paxil (paroxetine), Prozac (fluoxetine), or Zoloft (sertraline). They've been widely studied, and they're considered less likely to cause dependence in those who take them.

These medications do take a bit of time to start working. You probably won't feel relief from your symptoms immediately, but it's important to stick with it and keep taking the correct amount of medi-

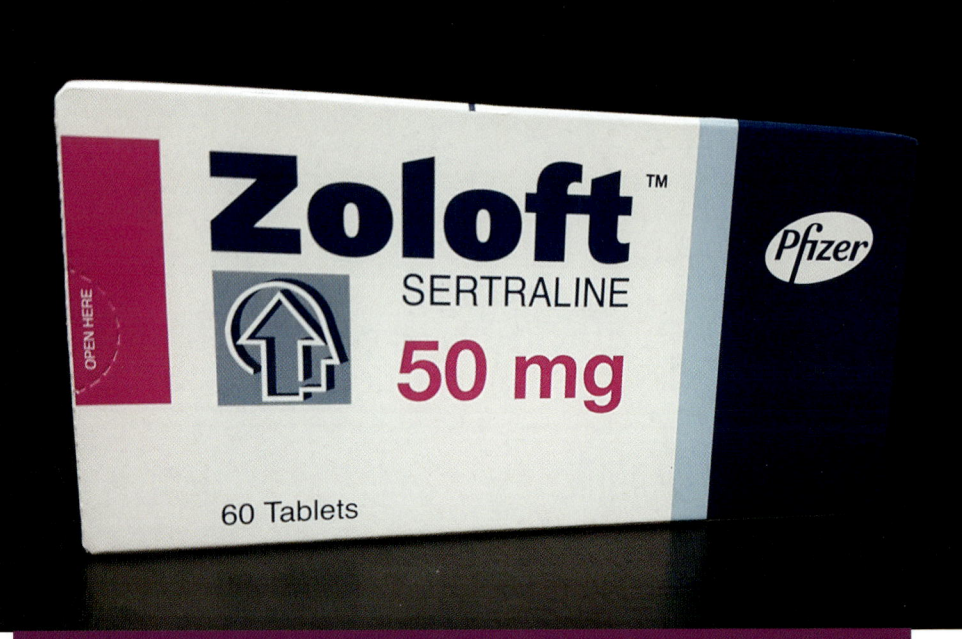

A doctor may prescribe a selective serotonin reuptake inhibitor (SSRI) such as Zoloft for you to take. It's very important to follow their instructions on how much to take and when.

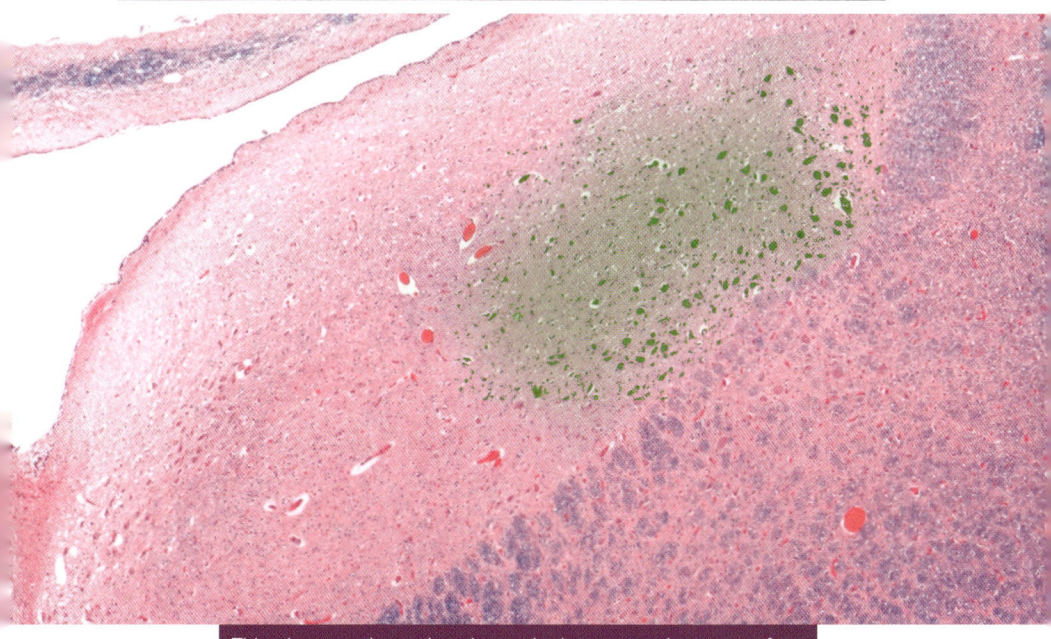

This close-up photo also shows the locus coeruleus part of the brain. Tricyclic antidepressants (TCAs) target this area.

cation. In about four to six weeks, you should begin to notice a difference.

SSRIs have more limited side effects than some other medications, but it's still important to pay attention to them. Always take only your prescribed amount of medication and don't take any other medication with it without your doctor's OK. If mild side effects don't go away after a few weeks, tell your doctor.

Another type of medication sometimes used for anxiety are antidepressants called tricyclic antidepressants (TCAs). They're often used for anxiety disorders, although they've become less popular because of the success of SSRIs. TCAs also block the uptake of serotonin in the brain, as well as the neurotransmitter norepinephrine. They target the locus coeruleus, the part of the brain that causes panic attacks. They're often prescribed under the names Elavil (amitriptyline), Adapin and Sinequan (doxepin), Tofranil (imipramine), and others.

MAO inhibitors (also known as MAOIs) are antidepressants too. They affect the neurotransmitters norepinephrine, serotonin, and dopamine. They're not prescribed as frequently these days. They can have many side effects depending on the things a

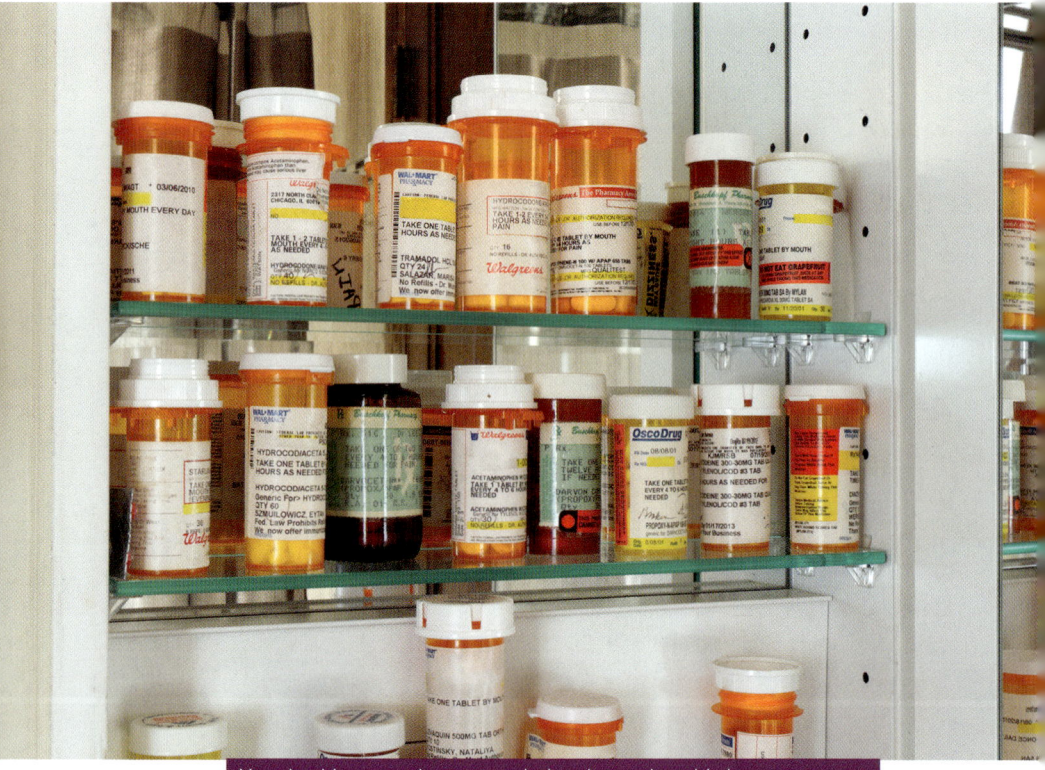

You should never take a prescription drug unless it's been prescribed just for you. Never take someone's else prescription.

person eats or drinks, and a number of other medications don't combine well with them.

Benzodiazepines are also used to help anxiety. These minor tranquilizers tend to act much more quickly, so they're also abused more. They target gamma-aminobutyric acid (GABA) receptors in the brain to make people relax. They're often prescribed under the names Ativan (lorazepam), Klonopin (clonazepam), Valium (diazepam), and Xanax (alprazolam). They're used on a more limited basis, but people must be very careful not to become dependent on them.

BENZODIAZEPINES AND ABUSE

While benzodiazepines such as Xanax can be very useful in managing the worst symptoms of anxiety and panic disorder, there are also dangers to these medications. Even though you can take them legally with a prescription, you can become reliant on them. Some people take more of their medication than they should or take benzodiazepines without a prescription. This can be very dangerous.

Today, many teenagers are becoming dependent on this type of prescription drug, sometimes called benzos. Taking too much can make a person black out and lose time, during which they have no memory of events. Combining benzos with alcohol or other drugs is particularly dangerous, but many teens do it. This can be deadly. While some people think benzos are a

(continued on the next page)

(continued from the previous page)

safer alternative to drugs such as opioids and heroin, they can be every bit as dangerous.

Even if you have a prescription for Xanax or another benzodiazepine, you can become used to the drug over time and need to take more and more for relief. Never increase your dosage without advice from a doctor. Never decrease it abruptly either—withdrawal can cause seizures or death.

If you have a problem with benzos, or you think a friend has a problem, talk to a trusted adult about what to do. You can break this addiction.

You can also call the U.S. Substance Abuse and Mental Health Services Administration (SAMHSA) national helpline at 1-800-662-HELP.

NO CURE-ALL

Medications can be a big help in dealing with panic and anxiety. It can give people the relief and distance from their anxiety and panic that makes it more possible to learn to deal with it. When you're not terrified of the possibility of a panic attack, you can learn to deal with it in a calmer way and manage it with other techniques.

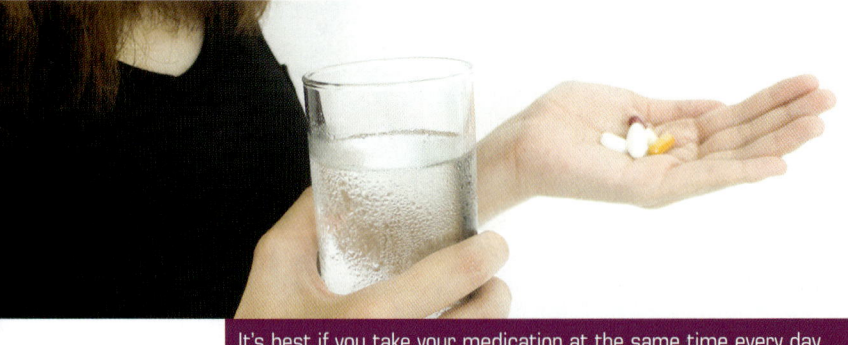

It's best if you take your medication at the same time every day.

However, there are limitations. It can take time for medication to work, and it can take time to find the right type and balance of medication. You have to take great care with many anxiety drugs. Also, relying simply on medication without learning ways to deal with your anxiety on your own doesn't ultimately help. Fortunately, there are techniques that can help you do so.

MYTHS AND FACTS ABOUT PANIC ATTACKS

- **MYTH #1:** Panic attacks are a sign of weakness. I should be able to manage this on my own.

- **FACT #1:** Everyday anxiety and nervousness are normal. Repeated and uncontrollable panic attacks are not. They're very scary, and there's nothing wrong with getting help for them. In fact, it's a brave thing to do. It's not weakness. It's an illness that can be treated.

- **MYTH #2:** I'll have to deal with panic attacks for the rest of my life.

- **FACT #2:** With some combination of lifestyle changes, medication, and therapy, you can successfully manage panic attacks.

- **MYTH #3:** You can die from a panic attack.

- **FACT #3:** Panic attacks are scary, but they can't hurt you—even though it often feels as though they can. Many of the symptoms of a panic attack make people think they're having a heart attack, but they're not the same thing.

CHAPTER 6

HOW TO FIND HELP

You may be reluctant to seek help for your panic attacks and anxiety. Many people are. However, when anxiety interferes with your life so much that you can't carry on your normal activities on a daily basis, you really do need professional help.

Think of it this way: People who are ill or injured go to see doctors to get help. Why should mental issues be any different? You wouldn't expect a person to be strong enough to heal a broken leg on their own, would you? But people often seem to think that someone should be able to manage anxiety without help.

If you suffer panic attacks or anxiety or are unable to overcome your phobias, you need professional help. This doesn't always mean a psychiatrist. Since anxiety disorders can be the result of medical conditions or chemical changes in your brain, it makes sense to have your primary care physician check you out before thinking that the trouble is purely an anxiety disorder.

A primary care doctor will work to determine possible physical causes of anxiety. That may entail

HOW TO FIND HELP 79

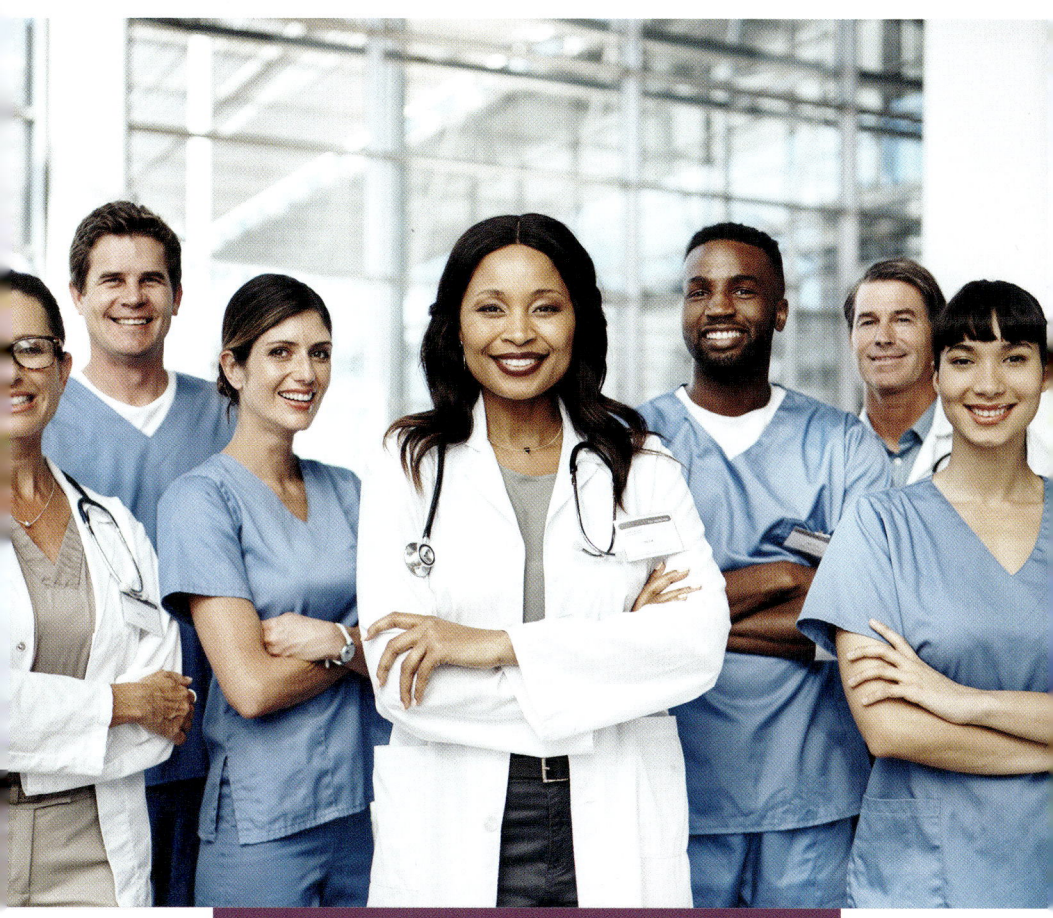

There are many kinds of mental health professionals that can help you learn what to do next about panic attacks and anxiety.

blood work, X-rays, and a thorough physical exam. They will probably ask about your family history as well, so know ahead of time if any of your relatives have certain health issues, including mental health issues. If the doctor rules out physical problems, they may refer you to a mental health professional for treatment.

MENTAL HEALTH PROFESSIONALS

Mental health professionals include psychiatrists, psychologists, clinical social workers, licensed professional counselors, and clinical nurses. Psychiatrists are the only ones who are also medical doctors. They can therefore prescribe medication, although others may also be able to do so based on their training and regulations in their state.

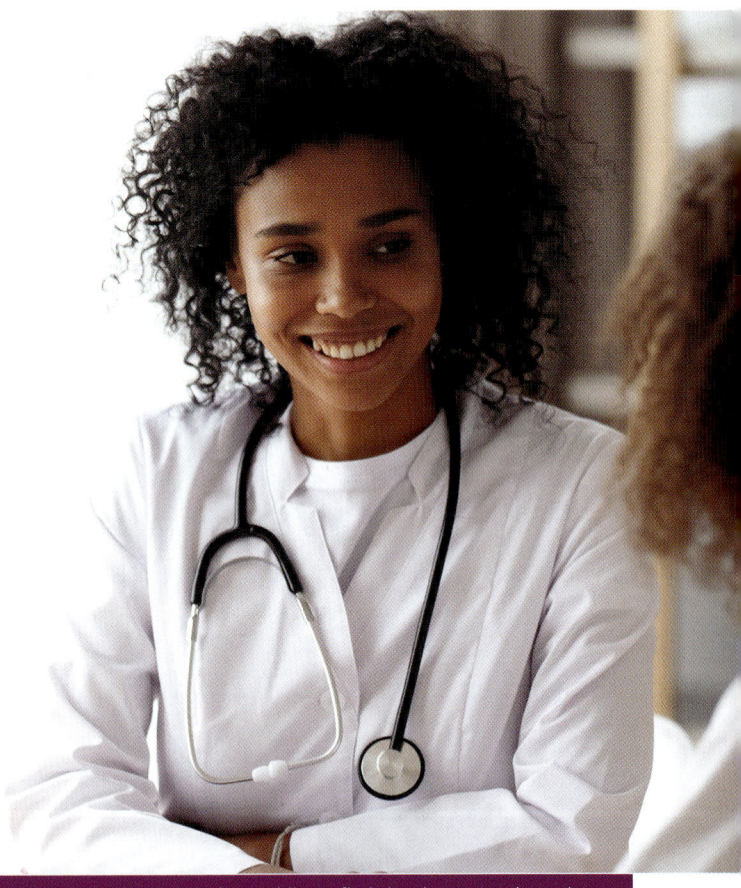

Just like with medications, it might take a while to find the doctor or therapist who's right for you. It's important that you be able to trust them and talk to them.

However, a visit to a psychiatrist's office may be costly. If an undiagnosed medical condition is clouding the picture, the psychiatrist might be quicker at spotting it, but you don't necessarily have to see a psychiatrist to get quality care. Often psychologists and social workers refer their clients who need medication to psychiatrists with whom they have a working relationship.

Psychologists have a doctoral degree. They're not medical doctors, but they have undergone a course of study for several years and have experience in a clinical setting. They're often knowledgeable about testing and can both administer and assess psychological tests.

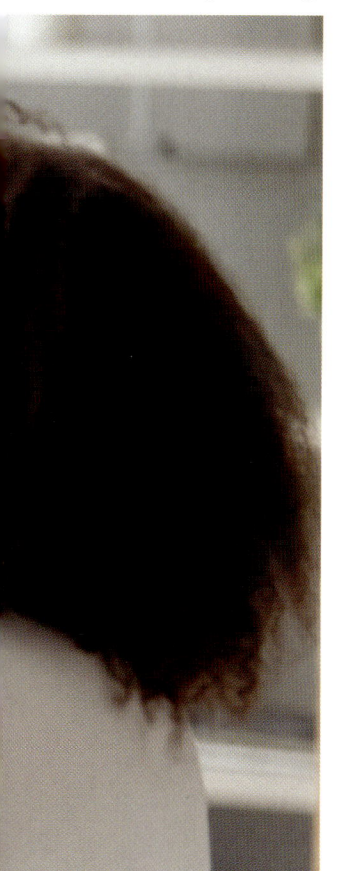

Clinical social workers may have either a master's degree or a doctorate degree in social work. They tend to provide most of the services to clients in mental health settings. They're also slightly less costly than psychologists and definitely less expensive than psychiatrists.

Psychiatric nurses, or clinical nurses, are also good choices because of their familiarity with medications and physical disorders. They're registered nurses with an advanced degree (usually a master's degree) in counseling.

No matter what the degree or title, all therapists are bound by the same basic set of ethics. They're not allowed to threaten or coerce you. If that ever happens, you have the right to stop services immediately. Tell a trusted adult. You may be able to report the therapist to the licensing board.

Likewise, therapists should not spend your time discussing their own problems (unless there is a connection) or asking you to do them favors. Therapy is a business relationship. Becoming friends with your therapist alters that business relationship and is unethical.

To some extent, therapists are supposed to keep what you tell them confidential. However, if you're younger than 18, confidentiality is a little different.

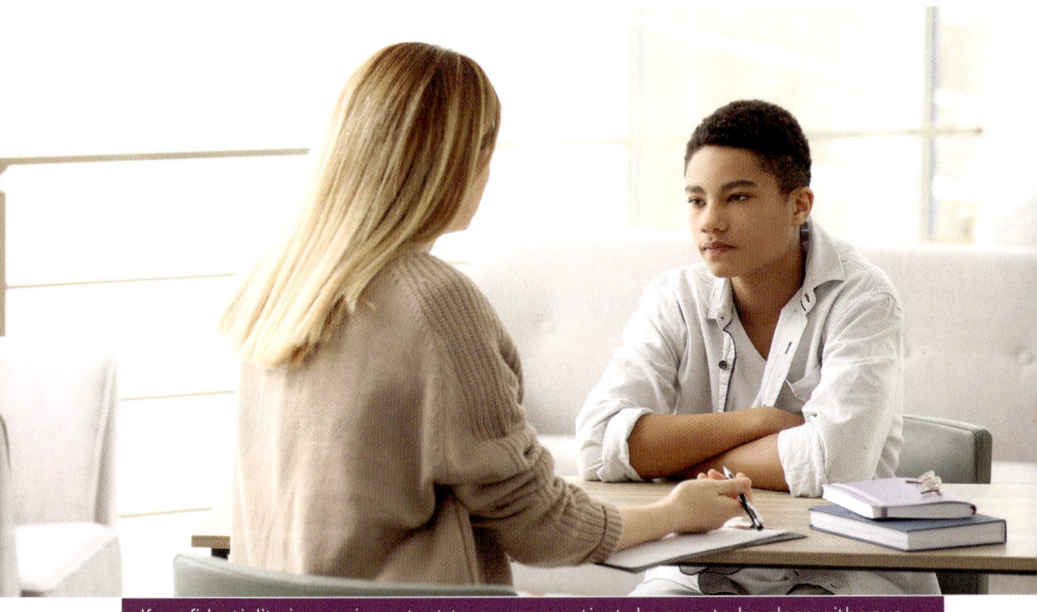

If confidentiality is very important to you as a patient, be sure to be clear with your therapist. They should be able to talk with you about it honestly and openly.

CONFIDENTIALITY FOR MINORS

If you're a minor (younger than 18), the usual rules of confidentiality with a therapist are likely limited a bit more than they are with an adult, at least when your parents or guardians are involved. Most minors don't have a legal right to privacy from their parents. However, for therapy to work, the person in therapy needs to be able to talk freely. That considered, some mental health professionals ask their patients' parents to agree to confidentiality rules before they'll talk to a new patient. After their patients have started treatment, the therapist may ask a patient to consent before they'll tell their parents certain things. Many rules vary by state. In some states, people as young as 12 can consent to mental health treatment. In other states, their parents or guardians must consent for them.

Minors still generally have the right of confidentiality with people other than their parents or guardians. Their therapists can't tell third parties about anything they say. This includes employers and others. Some states, including California, also give minors additional privacy rights.

However, if a therapist has a reason to believe a young person is in danger, they're often legally bound to report it to authorities. They must also report it if they believe their patient will harm themselves or others.

If you're seeing a new therapist, you, your parents or guardians, and the therapist should sit down together and discuss confidentiality rules and what all of you expect.

OTHER KINDS OF HELP

Support groups may be helpful for people with anxiety disorders. There, participants may learn how others with anxiety have managed their disorders. Support groups may or may not be run by professionals. Sometimes, people start a group to get together with others like themselves. They share advice on what strategies have worked for them and which therapists were most helpful. Most of these groups are not closed, meaning that people can join and drop out as they choose. It's helpful to have a professional therapist guide treatment, but it can be good to be able to talk to others who share your symptoms.

On the other side of things, sometimes anxiety can be so disabling that it requires hospitalization. Inpatient treatment is considered only when a person is thought to be a danger to themselves or others or if they're unable to meet their everyday needs. This may happen if someone with anxiety has suicidal thoughts. They may be hospitalized for treatment until they're no longer in danger.

Sometimes people are hospitalized so they can undergo more extensive testing. When physical disorders are suspected as the cause of anxiety, a patient may be hospitalized while the physical cause is being diagnosed.

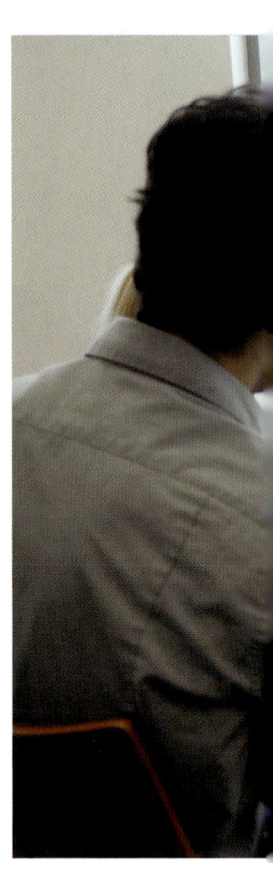

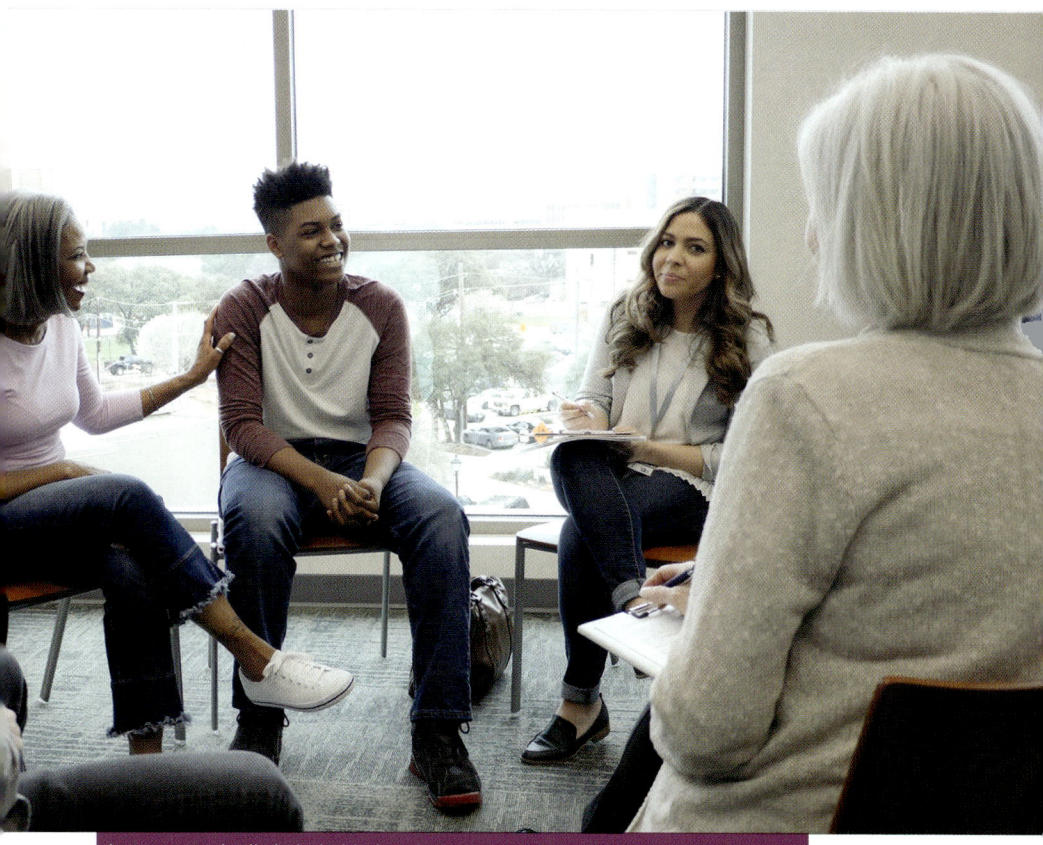

It may sound a little intimidating, but support groups can help people by introducing them to others dealing with the same issues and problems.

IT'S OK
Needing professional help to manage your anxiety is not a crime, nor is it something to be ashamed of. Anxiety disorders are complicated. Some people just need a little help to figure things out. Others need some level of professional help to learn how to manage. However you deal with your anxiety is the "right" way as long as it helps you to gain control over your symptoms.

CHAPTER 7

LIVING WITH ANXIETY AND STRESS

Even if you don't have panic disorder or another anxiety disorder, there may be many stressful situations in your life. The good news is that you can learn ways to handle these situations. If you understand how stress can create anxiety and you can effectively manage your reaction to that stress, you're less likely to develop an anxiety disorder. If you already have an anxiety disorder, you can learn more effective ways to manage your stress.

TRY RELAXATION TECHNIQUES

You can practice relaxation techniques to calm yourself and learn how to solve problems so that small issues don't grow into big ones. Practice tensing and relaxing all the muscles of your body. Start with your hand. Make a fist and clench as hard as you can. Hold that position for a few seconds, then release it. Relax your hand and wiggle your fingers to loosen it even more. Next, tense the muscles in your forearm. Try to do this without tensing your hand again. You want to isolate each body part as you tense and relax it. Hold the tensed position long enough to register how it feels. Then release and shake it loose. Progress up the arm, tensing, holding, and releasing.

Move on to the other hand and arm, then to the shoulders and neck. Next, tense and release your feet and move up your legs to your lower back, always tensing, holding, and releasing. Do these exercises when you can, preferably at night, because they'll relax you and prepare you for sleep. Take your time. If you don't have the time you need to do them all, spend a few minutes working on a specific part at a time.

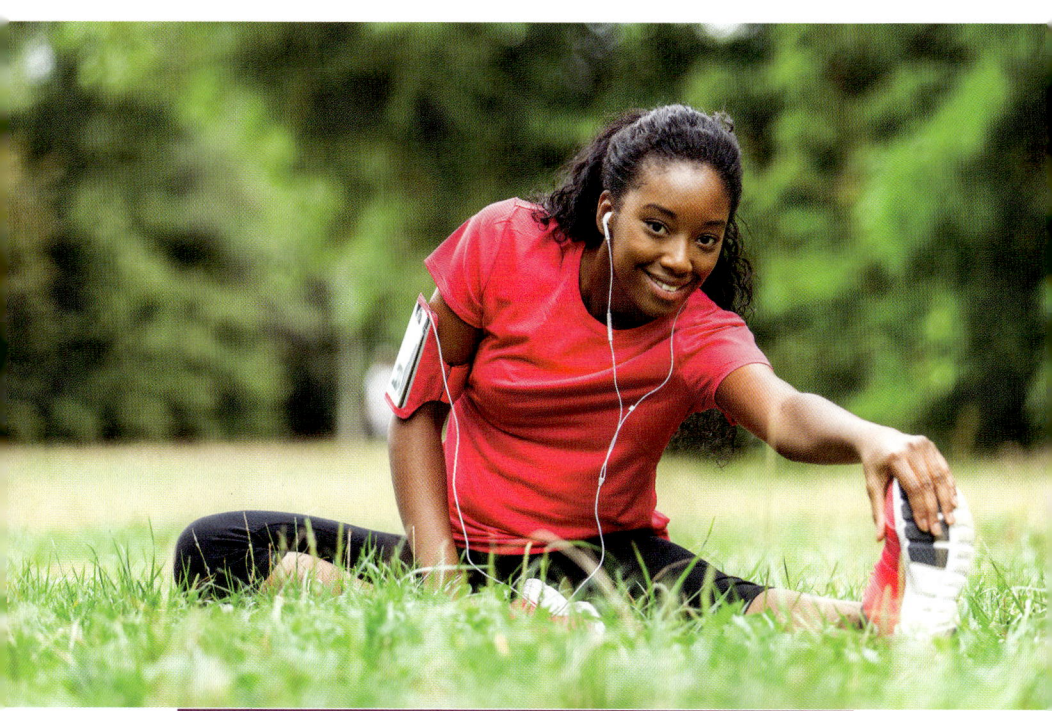

Stretching and other relaxation techniques can help you with anxiety.

Learn to control your breathing. Usually, most people breathe correctly, letting their abdomen expand and contract with each breath. This is called belly breathing. When stressed, however, people start panicking and tend to breathe more quickly and more shallowly. The chest rises and falls with each breath, indicating that the lungs are not expanding sufficiently to pull in oxygen and fully expel carbon dioxide. One of the quickest ways to relax yourself is to slow your breathing. Concentrate on the rise and fall of your abdomen. Push out your stomach, not your chest, and take the time to empty your lungs fully.

DO THINGS THAT CALM YOU

Life can be very stressful, but people need time to relax every day, not just once in a while. Try to plan for downtime each day. During this time, don't do anything but relax. You can also do things that relax you, such as creating art, watching television, listening to music or the sounds of nature, or reading for fun. Downtime allows you to rest so that you don't accumulate stresses from day to day.

You can also eliminate some things that lead to the opposite of calm. Caffeine is a stimulant. It can make people feel jittery and irritable. Reducing caffeine means reducing the amount of coffee, tea, and soda you drink, the amount of chocolate you eat, and the number of medications you take that contain caffeine. Nicotine, found in cigarettes, is another stimulant to avoid.

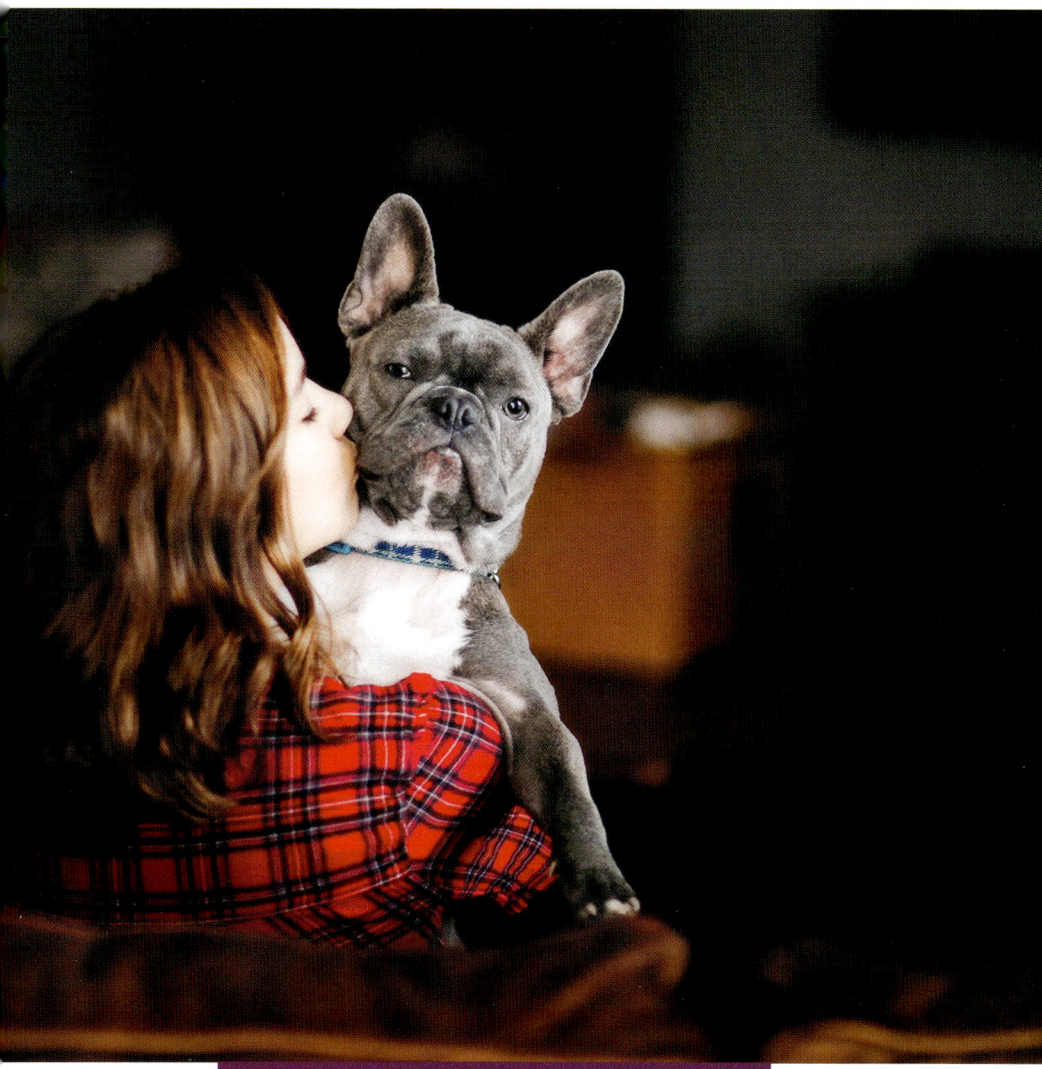

If you can, getting a pet can help with stress and anxiety. They give you something else to think about.

Developing an exercise routine can actually allow you to relax. This doesn't mean that you have to work out for hours each day. Simply taking a brisk walk for 30 minutes each day can help. In fact, scientists have discovered that the best measure for guarding against stress is regular exercise.

SET LIMITS AND STAND UP FOR YOURSELF

There are four main ways that a person can behave in relation to others. They can be aggressive, placing their own needs above anyone else's. They can be passive-aggressive, acting unintentionally in aggressive ways. They can be submissive, placing others' needs ahead of their own. Finally, they can be assertive, considering both their needs and the needs of others. An assertive person neither violates another person's space nor tolerates violation of their own space.

When people are assertive, they show respect both for themselves and others. Sometimes you'll want to say no when someone asks you for something. If you relent and say yes, you might feel angry at the person for putting you in that situation and at yourself for not saying what you really felt. Unresolved anger can lead to depression and, sometimes, aggression. When you say no and mean it, you show respect for yourself. You also stave off any anxious feelings about the situation and the people involved.

Setting limits goes along with saying no. People, especially family members, may sometimes push you to do more than you want to do, or they give you unsolicited advice. Set limits by determining the boundaries of your relationship. When someone oversteps that boundary, recognize it and assert yourself. People don't have the right to run your life unless you give them that right.

It's also important to learn how to stand up for yourself and express anger in an appropriate way. It's not enough just to recognize that you're angry, although that's a starting point. People can explode and then hurt others when they're angry, and that's just as inappropriate as holding in anger and ending up with a tension headache.

Learning to deal with anger begins with recognizing when you're angry, with whom you're angry, and why you're angry. Once you realize that you're angry (perhaps thanks to signs such as clenched teeth, a churning stomach, or a tension headache), consider who can change that situation, and then clarify the situation that needs to be changed.

Sometimes you might feel too angry to talk to the other person. When that happens, either try to calm yourself in order to gain perspective on the situation, or wear yourself out by exercising, cleaning, or playing a sport. The goal is to give yourself time to calm down and think more clearly. Taking your anger out by aggression, even to inanimate objects, is not a good thing. It doesn't calm you down; often it increases your anger.

It's OK to tell someone you're angry. Telling someone your feelings is far better than exploding from anger or holding them inside. However, try to look beyond the anger to the feelings underneath. These feelings are often ones of hurt, shame, or envy. Be prepared for the other person to have a different view of the situation. Listen if they present it, because you might discover that your view of the situation was not entirely accurate. Different solutions might present themselves. Anger itself doesn't cause more stress. The way people react to anger is the problem. If you're honest with your feelings and present them assertively (not aggressively), you stand to reduce your stress, not make it worse.

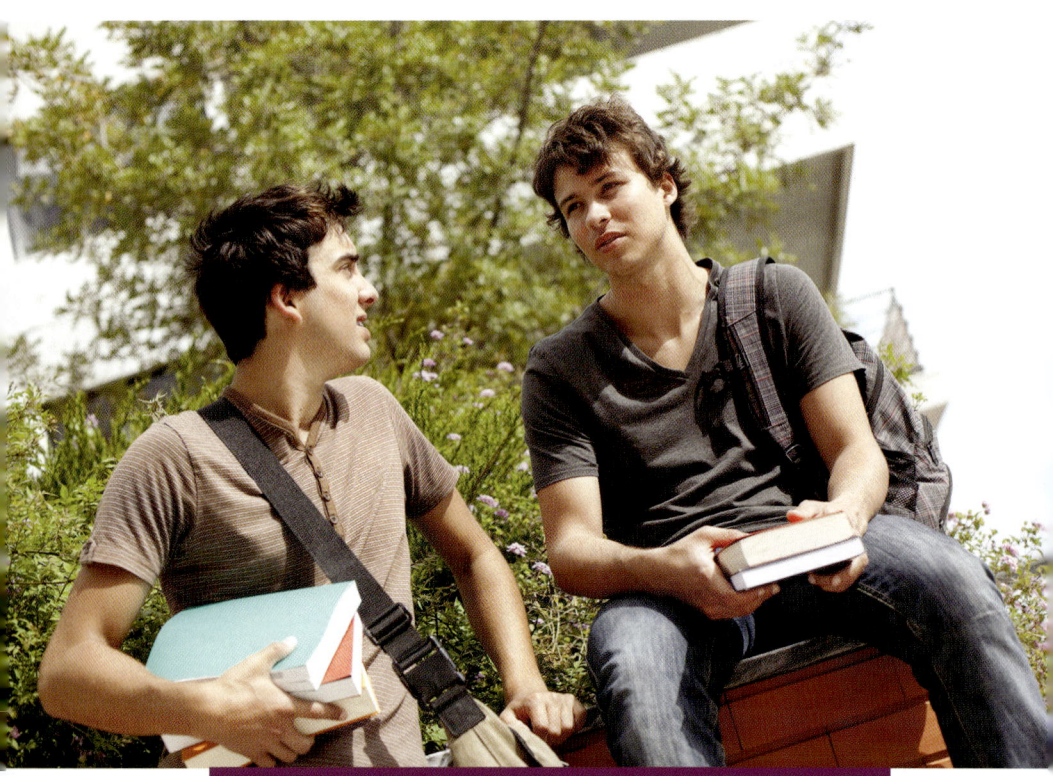

It's important to talk about and acknowledge your feelings, even when it's uncomfortable. Holding things in can just make it all worse.

TOXIC "FRIENDS"

It's good to spend time with your friends, right? That should help you manage stress and anxiety. But what if your friends are helping cause your stress and anxiety? How can you handle that?

Sometimes people (don't call them friends—real friends don't act like this) can be toxic. They can cause you to think in negative ways about yourself and others. They might put you down or manipulate you. They might accuse you of things you didn't do and delight in causing drama. They might get angry when good things happen to you and try to punish you. This isn't healthy in any kind of relationship.

How can you deal with toxic "friends?" If you want to try to save the friendship, you can try to stand up to this behavior and be assertive. Sometimes people will back down if they realize you're really upset. You can also slowly pull back from the friendship and see if the person wants to know why. If they want you as a friend, they can change their ways.

But what if you lose these so-called friends when you stand up for yourself? You probably don't want to hear it, but you're really better off without them. Give it time and work to make new friends—and this time, pay careful attention to what you want in a friend. Real friends support you. They might tell you occasional truths you need to hear, but they don't put you down just to make you feel badly about yourself. They don't do it to other people either. They treat you with respect, and they're fun to be around. As you talk to new people, keep these things in mind.

A MATTER OF TIME

Trouble with managing your time can often lead to stress and then to anxiety. You might feel overwhelmed and a little desperate to get back on top of things again. Figure out what's most important and

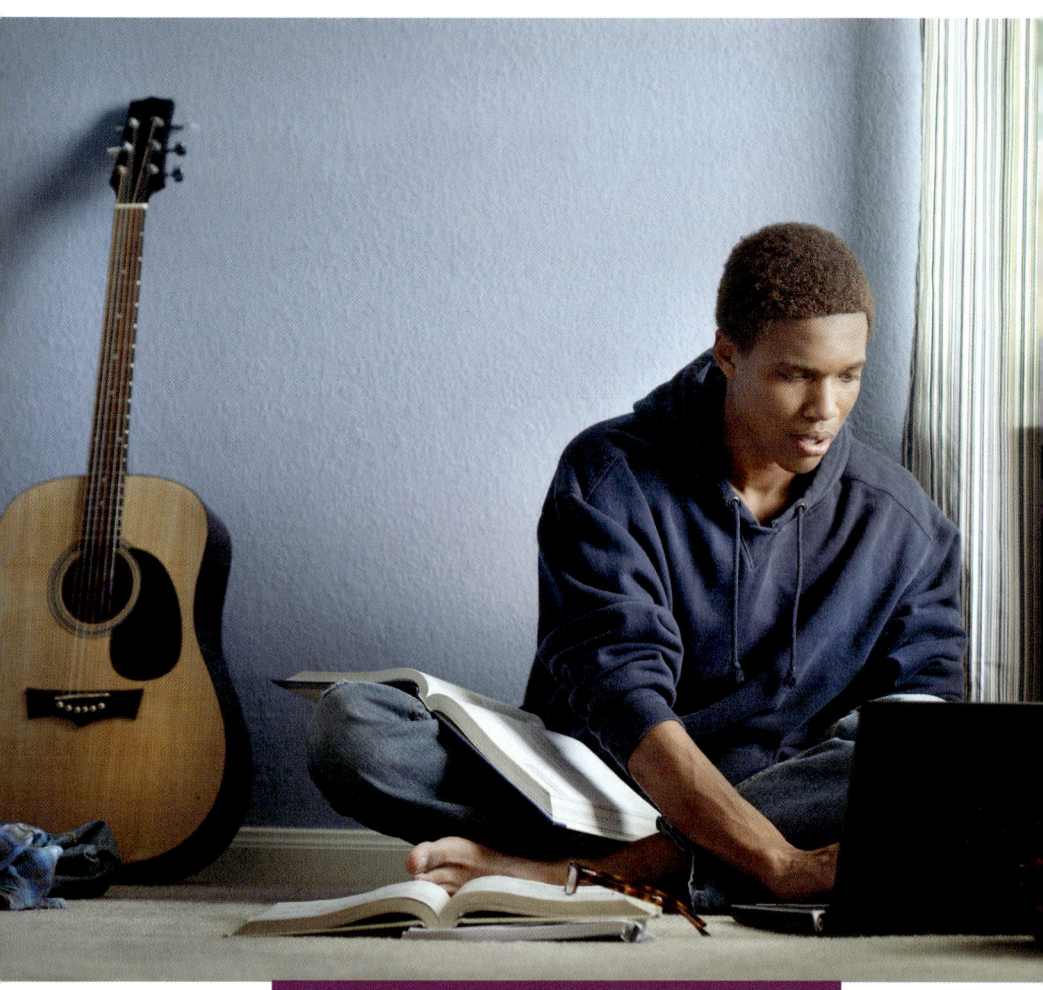

Making sure you manage your time well and have a chance to do things that relax you is key to dealing with anxiety.

LIVING WITH ANXIETY AND STRESS

what you need to get done first. Get that done, then work your way down your list. It might be tough to find time to do all the things you want to do. You might have to consider giving up something—a sport, a club, a job—if you can so that you're not spread too thin. There are only so many hours in a day. Make sure you can keep a little downtime in your schedule.

Sometimes lists can help people prioritize what they need to do. Try making lists with goals in the order of what you need to do. Don't try to do too much in one day. Try talking to your parents or a trusted teacher, coach, counselor, or friend about what you can pare down or put off. Your mental health is important!

GLOSSARY

adrenaline Hormone secreted by the adrenal glands that raises the blood pressure, causing the heart to pound and the senses to become alerted to the possibility of danger.

aggressive Disposed to dominate without regard for the feelings of others.

antidepressant Class of medication designed to reduce clinical depression.

behavioral reaction The actions a person takes in response to another person's actions.

benzodiazepines A group of drugs, minor tranquilizers often prescribed to alleviate panic attacks.

bruxism Grinding of the teeth, especially during stress.

cognitive distortion Mistaken beliefs about events that cause stress and the conviction that the worst will occur as a result.

cognitive reaction Way of thinking about anxiety that may actually increase the severity of anxiety.

defense mechanism Unconscious mental approach to a problem to try to resolve it.

displacement Transfer of anger against a powerful person to another person who poses no threat.

downtime A period of time specifically set aside for relaxation, without the need to accomplish any task.

exposure Act of putting oneself in actual contact with the object of a phobia.

insomnia Inability to fall asleep or stay asleep; it may have a physical or psychological basis.

obsessive-compulsive disorder Mental disorder involving the need to repeat a behavior, such as hand washing.

passive-aggressive Unconsciously disposed to act in a demanding way, without regard for the feelings of others.

phobia A long-lasting and irrationally strong fear of an object or a situation. A simple phobia is fear of a specific thing; social phobia refers to the fear of embarrassing oneself in public.

physiological Pertaining to a physical symptom of the body.

rationalization Application of rational motives to questionable behavior.

reaction formation Defense mechanism by which one credits oneself with good motives when the motives are actually negative.

regression Defense mechanism in which one reverts to an earlier, less stressful, period of life.

repression Defense mechanism in which one unconsciously forgets events.

stimulant Substance that causes a temporary increase in the function of the body or parts of the body.

submissive Having a tendency to give in to others, putting their concerns ahead of your own.

systematic desensitization Gradual elimination of fears by coming into repeated contact with the feared object.

ulcer An open sore in the stomach wall caused by excess production of stomach acids, sometimes as a result of stressful conditions.

FOR MORE INFORMATION

Anxiety and Depression Association of America
8701 Georgia Avenue, Suite 412
Silver Spring, MD 20910
(240) 485-1001
Website: www.adaa.org
This nonprofit organization is dedicated to the prevention, treatment, and cure of anxiety, depressive, obsessive-compulsive, and trauma-related disorders through education, practice, and research.

Anxiety Canada
811-402 West Prender Street
Vancouver, BC, Canada V6B 1T6
(604) 620-0744
Website: anxietycanada.org
This charity and nonprofit organization raises awareness about anxiety and supports access to proven research and treatment.

International OCD Foundation
P.O. Box 961029
Boston, MA 02196
(617) 973-5801
Website: iocdf.org
The mission of the foundation is to help those affected by obsessive-compulsive disorder and related disorders to live full and productive lives. Its aim is to increase access to effective treatment through research and training, foster a hopeful and supportive community for those affected by OCD and the professionals who treat them, and fight stigma surrounding mental health issues.

The Kim Foundation
11949 Q Street
Omaha, NE 68137
(402) 891-6911

Website: thekimfoundation.org
The foundation's mission is to serve as a supportive resource and compassionate voice for lives touched by mental illness and suicide. Its vision is a community free of suicide that embraces the importance of quality mental health services and prevention.

Mental Health America
500 Montgomery Street, Suite 820
Alexandria, VA 223114
(800) 969-6642
Website: www.mhanational.org
Mental Health America is the nation's leading community-based nonprofit dedicated to addressing the needs of those living with mental illness and to promoting the overall mental health of all.

National Alliance on Mental Illness (NAMI)
4301 Wilson Blvd., Suite 300
Arlington, VA 22203
(703) 524-7600
Website: www.nami.org
NAMI provides advocacy, education, support, and public awareness so that all individuals and families affected by mental illness can build better lives.

National Institute of Mental Health (NIMH)
Office of Science Policy, Planning, and Communication Branch
6001 Executive Boulevard, Room 6200, MSC 9663
Bethesda, MD 20892-9663
(866) 615-6464
Website: www.nimh.nih.gov
NIMH envisions a world in which mental illnesses are prevented and cured.

FOR FURTHER READING

Aman, Jodi. *Anxiety…I'm So Done with You: A Teen's Guide to Ditching Stress and Hardwiring Your Brain for Happiness.* New York, NY: Skyhorse Publishing, 2020.

Galanti, Regine. *Anxiety Relief for Teens: Essential CBT Skills and Mindfulness Practices to Overcome Anxiety and Stress.* New York, NY: Zeitgeist, 2020.

Huebner, Dawn. *Outsmarting Worry.* Philadelphia, PA: Jessica Kingsley Publishers, 2018.

Hutt, Rachel L. *Feeling Better: CBT Workbook for Teens.* Emeryville, CA: Althea Press, 2019.

Jain, Renee. *Superpowered: Transform Anxiety into Courage, Confidence, and Resilience.* New York, NY: Random House, 2020.

Ona, Patricia Zarita. *The Act Workbook for Teens with OCD.* London, UK: Jessica Kingsley Publishers, 2019

Riegel, Sophie. *Don't Tell Me to Relax! One Teen's Journey to Survive Anxiety and How You Can Too.* Oceanside, CA: Indie Books International, 2019.

Romain, Trevor, and Elizabeth Verdick. *Stress Can Really Get on Your Nerves! (Laugh and Learn)*. Minneapolis, MN: Free Spirit Publishing, 2018.

Sedley, Ben. *Stuff That Sucks: A Teen's Guide to Accepting What You Can't Change and Committing to What You Can*. Oakland, CA: Instant Help, an imprint of New Harbinger Publications, 2017.

Tompkins, Michael A. *My Anxious Mind: A Teen's Guide to Managing Anxiety and Panic*. Washington, DC: Magination Press, 2010.

INDEX

A
agoraphobia, 11, 24, 39, 40, 46, 47, 48

B
benzodiazepines, 75, 76

C
catastrophic thinking, 31, 57, 59

D
defense mechanisms, 50, 52, 53, 54, 64
depression, 10, 34, 43, 44, 49, 59, 90
dopamine, 10, 74

G
gamma-aminobutyric acid (GABA), 10, 75
generalized anxiety disorder (GAD), 34, 36

H
heart, 4, 8, 17, 29, 35, 36, 45, 46, 48, 63, 77
hyperventilation, 18, 62

I
irritable bowel syndrome (IBS), 6, 16, 17

L
locus coeruleus, 18, 19, 73, 74

M
MAO inhibitors (MAOIs), 74
muscles, 4, 45, 60, 62, 65, 66

N
National Alliance on Mental Illness (NAMI), 34
neurotransmitter, 10, 11, 12, 19, 20, 72, 74
nightmares and night terrors, 12, 13, 14, 15, 24
norepinephrine, 10, 19, 74

O
obsessive-compulsive disorder (OCD), 20, 21, 34, 41, 42, 43, 68

P
phobias, 24, 25, 26, 27, 34, 39, 40, 50, 56, 60, 62, 65, 66, 67, 68, 78
post-traumatic stress disorder (PTSD), 22, 24, 34, 38, 39

S
selective serotonin reuptake inhibitors (SSRIs), 72, 73
serotonin, 10, 19, 20, 72, 74
social phobias, 24, 26, 39, 40
stomach, 4, 6, 8, 17, 27, 36, 44, 91

T
trauma, 14, 22, 23, 38, 39
tricyclic antidepressants (TCAs), 73

ABOUT THE AUTHOR

Verity Miller is a writer and editor who was first diagnosed with panic disorder and anxiety when she was 19, after panic attacks started hitting during her first year of college. She hopes this book will help young people learn more about these conditions and that it's OK to get help for them. Miller enjoys reading, cooking, gaming, and traveling. She lives with her spouse and kids in New York State.

CREDITS

Photo Credits: Cover, FluxFactory/ E+/Getty Images; Cover, pp. 1-104 LUMIKK555/Shutterstock.com; Cover, pp. 1-104 Filin84/Shutterstock.com; p. 5 ljubaphoto/ E+/Getty Images; p. 7 G-Stock Studio/Shutterstock.com; p. 9 Kmatta/Moment/Getty Images; p. 10 https://commons.wikimedia.org/wiki/File:Cell_GABA_Receptor.png; p. 13 PhotoAlto/Frederic Cirou/PhotoAlto Agency RF Collections/Getty Images; p. 15 Antonio Guillem/Shutterstock.com; p. 16 Jirattawut Domrong/Shutterstock.com; p. 19 https://commons.wikimedia.org/wiki/File:Locus_ceruleus_-_high_mag.jpg; pp. 21, 55, 80 zkes/Shutterstock.com; p. 23 Yiannis Papadimitriou/Shutterstock.com; p. 25 Apexphotos/Moment/Getty Images; p. 28 Peter Dazeley/The Image Bank/Getty Images; p. 30 Klaus Vedfelt/ DigitalVision/Getty Images; p. 33 Stuart Jenner/Shutterstock.com; p. 35 anchai Pundej /EyeEm/Getty Images; p. 37 Photographee.eu/Shutterstock.com; p. 38 SDI Productions/E+/Getty Images; p. 42 Andrey_Popov/Shutterstock.com; p. 44 Maskot/Getty Images; p. 47 Jasmin Merdan/Moment/Getty Images; p. 49 SpeedKingz/Shutterstock.com; p. 51 SolStock/E+/Getty Images; p. 53 Halfpoint/Shutterstock.com; p. 56 Pixel-Shot/Shutterstock.com; p. 61 David Trood/ DigitalVision/Getty Images; p. 63 Song_about_summer/Shutterstock.com; p. 64 Housh/Shutterstock.com; p. 71 Portrait Image Asia/Shutterstock.com; p. 72 Omeletzz/Shutterstock.com; p. 73 https://commons.wikimedia.org/wiki/File:Locus_coeruleus_highlighted.jpg; p. 74 Kimberly Boyles/Shutterstock.com; p. 76 memorisz/Shutterstock.com; p. 79 Cecilie_Arcurs/E+/Getty Images; p. 82 New Africa/Shutterstock.com; p. 85 SDI Productions/E+/Getty Images; p. 87 Samuel Borges Photography/Shutterstock.com; p. 89 Rebecca Nelson/ Photodisc/Getty Images; p. 92 Helder Almeida/Shutterstock.com; p. 94 Terry Vine/ DigitalVision/Getty Images; p. 95 Tutatama lm/Shutterstock.com.